the
yoga face

Annelise Hagen

AVERY *a member of Penguin Group (USA) Inc., New York*

the
yoga face

Eliminate Wrinkles with
the Ultimate Natural Facelift

Published by the Penguin Group
Penguin Group (USA) Inc., 375 Hudson Street, New York, New York 10014, USA • Penguin Group (Canada),
90 Eglinton Avenue East, Suite 700, Toronto, Ontario M4P 2Y3, Canada (a division of Pearson Penguin Canada Inc.) •
Penguin Books Ltd, 80 Strand, London WC2R 0RL, England • Penguin Ireland, 25 St Stephen's Green, Dublin 2,
Ireland (a division of Penguin Books Ltd) • Penguin Group (Australia), 250 Camberwell Road, Camberwell,
Victoria 3124, Australia (a division of Pearson Australia Group Pty Ltd) • Penguin Books India Pvt Ltd,
11 Community Centre, Panchsheel Park, New Delhi–110 017, India • Penguin Group (NZ), 67 Apollo Drive,
Rosedale, North Shore 0745, Auckland, New Zealand (a division of Pearson New Zealand Ltd) •
Penguin Books (South Africa) (Pty) Ltd, 24 Sturdee Avenue, Rosebank, Johannesburg 2196, South Africa

Penguin Books Ltd, Registered Offices: 80 Strand, London WC2R 0RL, England

Most Avery books are available at special quantity discounts for bulk purchase for sales promotions, premiums, fund-raising,
and educational needs. Special books or book excerpts also can be created to fit specific needs. For details, write Penguin Group
(USA) Inc. Special Markets, 375 Hudson Street, New York, NY 10014.

Library of Congress Cataloging-in-Publication Data
Hagen, Annelise.
The yoga face: eliminate wrinkles with the ultimate natural facelift
p.   cm.
Includes bibliographical references and index.
ISBN 978-1-58333-277-1
1. Facial exercises.   2. Hatha yoga.   3. Beauty, Personal.   I. Title.
RA778.H34   2007   2007008434
613.7'046—dc22

Printed in the United States of America
9   10

BOOK DESIGN BY NICOLE LAROCHE

Neither the publisher nor the author is engaged in rendering professional advice or services to the individual reader. The ideas,
procedures, and suggestions in this book are not intended as a substitute for consulting with a physician. All matters regarding
health require medical supervision. If you have any health problems or medical conditions, consult with your physician before
undertaking any of the instructions in this book. Neither the author nor the publisher shall be liable or responsible for any loss
or damage allegedly arising from any information or suggestion in this book.

The recipes in this book are to be followed exactly as written. The publisher is not responsible for specific health or allergy
conditions that may require medical supervision. The publisher is not responsible for any adverse reactions to the recipes in
this book.

While the author has made every effort to provide accurate telephone numbers and Internet addresses at the time of publication,
neither the publisher nor the author assumes any responsibility for errors, or for changes that occur after publication. Further, the
publisher does not have any control over and does not assume any responsibility for author or third-party websites or their
content.

Contents

Introduction

Imagine you are in a busy metropolitan center at rush hour. Everywhere you look, you see athletic bodies, dressed in designer suits and body-hugging oufits. But look above the neckline. Do these fit physiques sport equally firm faces? What you may see instead are wrinkles and bags: the indelible marks of stress and lack of exercise misshaping the canvas of the face.

The Yoga Face operates on a simple principle: The muscles of the face are no different from the muscles in the rest of your body. If you don't exercise the muscles below the neck, they become weak and flabby; the same goes for the muscles of the face. The Yoga Face is a set of exercises and stretches that provides these all-important muscles the same youthful tightening and toning that going to the gym offers below the neck.

When a muscle "works," it becomes firmer. When a muscle has something to "work against" (i.e., resistance), it becomes stronger. A sedentary muscle will gain fat and lose tone, and in the face, this will manifest itself as sagging and drooping. While the facial muscles are smaller, they are still muscles, like any other in your body. They need to lift, expand, and contract, in order to stay healthy, fit, and beautiful. Like the other muscles of the body, they need to receive lots of fresh, life-giving oxygen. And like any other muscle, they can be trained.

I have been teaching yoga for eight years in some of the top fitness clubs and yoga studios in New York City. Over the years, I gradually became aware of something interesting—and disconcerting—in my classes. My student yogis flowed through intricate sequences with ease. Following my cues, they breathed in perfect unison with their actions. They performed complex *asanas* (yoga poses) with steadiness and grace. The rooms were filled with youthful and vibrant practitioners.

Yet when I looked at many of their faces, I could see the telltale signs of strain and stress: the young woman with the dancer's physique contorted her face into a scowl; the toned fellow across the room furrowed his brow in concentration. Meanwhile, another woman held a pose with clenched jaw and pursed lips. It was almost as if they were taking all the nervous energy the poses were releasing from their bodies and pouring it into their faces. I saw that I had been paying much more attention to the health of the body below the neck than above it. I began telling people to relax their faces, to exhale on a sigh, or to unclench their jaws, and I saw that as they released their faces, they derived more benefit from the poses, and also began to look more youthful!

I began to wonder if the same exercise principles that worked for the body could also work for the face—with some modification. While weights obviously were not practical, why couldn't facial muscles derive the benefits of exercise: performing repetitive motion to burn off fat; flushing the cells, muscles, and tissues with oxygenated blood; and countering habitual emotional tendencies that lead to gripping and clenching, and by extension, wrinkles?

I started experimenting with yoga postures, developing a class that would specifically address anti-aging for the face. I wanted to help transform the faces of my students the way I had seen their bodies transform. In addition, I began an in-depth study of facial anatomy, and also began a regime of exercise for my own facial muscles.

At a yoga studio I was affiliated with, I developed a workshop that focused on yoga poses that were known to be anti-aging and calming. I blended the poses yogis call "restorative" with some facial toning work I had learned in my vocal training as an actress. These exercises worked with jaw tension and training the lips, tongue, and teeth for expression. They were effective, improving skin and muscle tone in the face, and performing them often left me with a bit of a lactic acid "burn" like running or lifting weights did in my other body parts. As I practiced them along with the yoga poses, I got excited by the rapid diminishing of signs of aging on my face.

While experimenting with this work, I remembered other vocal exercises I had learned when I was in my twenties and working as a stage actress. Some of these were specifically designed to work with breathing capacity, increasing oxygen flow in and out of the body. These exercises were energizing, and you could see the benefits on the surface of the skin immediately. Many of the vocal exercises were designed to release tension from the jaw and the face.

I realized as I performed my facial "gymnastics" that perhaps fifty percent of the appearance of aging in the face was a result of tension. In both myself and others I observed, the long-term repeated facial patterns of tension embedded on the face in the form of wrinkles, and in the moment they showed up as unflattering and involuntary scowls, frowns, and creases. After this realization, the evidence grew—or maybe I had just become more aware of something that had been going on for a long time—and I would find myself suddenly reflected in a shop window, scowling when I was perfectly happy, or I'd see myself in the reflection of a subway door, frowning in a moment of concentration. But just a few moments of facial exercises released the mask of worry, fear, and anger. By practicing conscious relaxation, in combination with the facial exercises, I had found a one-two punch to counter the signs of facial aging.

This program has had a profound effect on my self-confidence and sense of hope for the future of my skin. In my twenties, I had wantonly played in the sun, sans hat or sunscreen. I had consumed caffeine and sugar liberally. I had burned the midnight oil—all without much thought to the condition of my skin. But the clock began to catch up. Many skin experts will confirm this: the damage we create from sun exposure, poor diet, and lack of exercise up into our twenties usually doesn't show up on the skin as visible signs until our thirties. When this problem is coupled with the loss of collagen and elastin (the proteins that help our connective tissues stay firm and resilient) that occurs as we age, it's no wonder many people wake up in their thirties to discover skin damage they hadn't known was there. On my thirty-third birthday, I found a worry line between my brows that didn't go away, even when I consciously relaxed. I also noticed discolorations and patches on my skin—what I thought were sunspots but may also have been signs of nutritional imbalance. Still, I persisted in blithely ignoring the warning signs most of the time. I thought there was no remedy for past damage done— as so many tomes on skin proclaim—only to become despondent when confronted with the ugly truth in a particularly candid snapshot. As I studied the photo, I thought, "Who is this person who bears only a fleeting resemblance to how I have pictured myself? That isn't my elderly aunt—that's *me!* Why don't the bags under my eyes know that I am a yoga teacher?" Meanwhile, as I was teaching my students the principles of acceptance and detachment, some of my teaching peers were getting facial work done. These people were preaching inner contentment, that the true source of happiness lies within. But off the record, they admitted to me they felt pressure to look youthful— that, in fact, their livelihoods depended on it. I knew of one yoga teacher who received regular lip injections! But I was concerned a measure such as that could possibly reduce my facial mobility—something I knew I didn't want to lose!

I was pursuing inner peace and calm but still debating a nip here and a tuck there. One of my colleagues, having just turned forty (and none too thrilled about it), got an eyelift. I was curious to see the results. After a few weeks of absence, she returned to work. Three thousand dollars later, her eyes did look a little smoother. But her palpably low self-esteem offset any positive effects of the surgery. She still looked depressed and critical of herself. And a year later, I saw that her anxiety had brought many of the lines she'd attempted to lift right back to her skin. So it's true, I mused to myself. If you don't change the behavior that led to the wrinkles to begin with, the habitual facial expressions that you unconsciously perform hundred of times throughout the day will etch themselves permanently. It's like people who get surgery to lose weight yet don't change their eating habits: it's the behavior, not the symptom, that causes the problem and that must be corrected!

I continued practicing my facial program at home in front of the mirror and on the yoga mat, as well as in classes with more and more of my yoga students. I thought to myself that I would try, as an experiment, whatever I could with the tools I already had to transform my face naturally. If all else failed, I would consider other methods. I was hoping the natural alternative would work, as I didn't want to defy my principles or dent my wallet. It was difficult at first, as training my facial muscles to isolate and resist gravity by using pressure from my fingertips was new and hard to master—but after a session, I would notice changes right away. The circulation traveled to my face, the glow increased, and the droops and shar-pei furrows decreased. The awareness I began to develop about my facial habits sometimes was upsetting—I never realized how much of an involuntary scowler I had become (although my mother has showed me pictures of myself as a one-year-old, resting my chin on my palm and frowning like a curmudgeon). But gradually, my facial appearance became new and improved. The techniques I was practicing were actually working!

I had discovered the answer for me, my colleagues, and for all people considering getting (or who have already had) work done. From my preliminary research and efforts, I taught a well-attended onetime workshop at a Manhattan yoga studio. The response was overwhelming. My students—women and men, old and young—seemed thrilled at finding the prospect of a positive and healthy solution to the signs of facial aging. The workshop blossomed into an ongoing weekly class at the New York Health & Racquet Club.

Working with the face took practice for all of us. We were clumsy mastering the willful control of the small facial muscles that heretofore had moved only involuntarily for most of us. But with practice we quickly became adept at isolating our facial muscles and voluntarily performing facial exercises. We all obtained noticeable results within weeks. The students looked and felt more youthful, more positive, more radiant, and therefore more attractive. They reported feeling powerful instead of feeling helpless. Those who were considering getting work done started realizing that they had options. They had found a safe, natural, and effective alternative by going to the root rather than staying on the surface.

Since these initial workshops, the Yoga Face has turned into one of the most sought-after classes in the highly competitive world of New York fitness. Over the last two years, I have been honing and refining the method constantly. Now, in response to overwhelming demand, I have culled all of these teachings into this first book on the Yoga Face. It really is the ultimate natural facelift.

The Yoga Face isn't a miracle cure (we all know how well those tend to work); rather, it is a results-oriented program that is as effective as the amount of work you put into it. With the Yoga Face, you can give your face a smoother and firmer appearance, and simultaneously improve your energy and mood. I cannot promise that you won't age, but I can assure you that if you practice these principles and exercises, you will be able to slow down the rate at which you age visibly. Along the way, you will gain some other yogic skills for destressing, detoxing, and purifying your body, mind, and spirit. You'll feel calm and serene on the inside, which will match how you look on the outside. The only surprise you'll encounter when catching your reflection in a busy street window or a candid snapshot will be one of delight.

chapter one

Regain Your Youth
with Facial Fitness

The face of a yogic sage is marvelous to behold: beaming, joyful, bright-eyed, full of love and compassion . . . and noticeably unlined. If you were to ask such a sage how old he is, you might well be shocked: even a ninety-year-old yogi can be remarkably smooth-skinned and wrinkle-free.

What is the key to his ageless condition? Is it the result of performing complicated, pretzel-like twists and arm balances? In actuality, many yogic sages don't do much of the physical practice of yoga at all. They spend a great deal more time in meditation, service, and study than in the yoga postures. Perhaps there is another yogic secret about youthfulness that the sages possess.

Now let's examine a thirty- or fortysomething American woman who is in great shape. This woman has a toned, muscular body: slim and glowing, she walks down the street confidently. She faithfully works out or takes yoga classes during the week, and the exercise makes her body lean, strong, and flexible. But check out her face and you may be surprised: she has bags under her eyes, her skin is dull, and her brow is puckered into an unattractive scowl. Isn't fitness supposed to make you look young?

These two examples reflect two very different lifestyles. The yogic sage reflects the traditional Indian spiritual approach. The woman has a more Western, modern lifestyle. Neither approach is better than the other, for they are each products of their particular culture and environment. The Eastern traditions of contemplation, introspection, and acceptance help create serenity. The Western approach is more active, emphasizing fitness over contemplation. The Western approach is often act first, reflect later—if at all.

Life in our modern Western society seems to focus on incessant activity, consumption, and rushing from point A to point B to accomplish these aims. We are constantly trying to find the time to slow down and see friends or family, or just get our basic needs and day-to-day tasks met. This produces a lot of stress, and is manifested by myriad stress-related diseases, such as high cholesterol, heart disease, addictive behaviors (smoking and excessive eating and drinking), and related illnesses (cancer, obesity, hypertension). In addition to showing up in the body, stress manifests almost instantly on the sensitive emotional mirror of the face.

Here in the West, even our approach to health has become an obsession. We seem to apply our manic work ethic to fitness. Many people now feel that if they don't work out daily, or at least three or four times a week, they are doomed to decay or atrophy. In some ways, the frenetic and incessant movement we all seem to engage in is just that: a denial of stillness, and its most final manifestation, death. At the very least, people fear that if they don't strenuously exercise their bodies in a punishing way, they will be too fat, or simply unattractive. I certainly have been one of those people. I have exhausted myself with intense exercise out of fear of gaining weight or being unattractive. Strangely, as I have relaxed and slowed down, I have gotten slimmer, less compulsive about eating and working out, and, yes, my face has relaxed and de-aged amazingly. In fact, since I started applying the Yoga Face principles to my life, my face seems to look younger, better rested, and more vibrant with each day.

Even the yoga currently popular in gyms and studios these days reflects our preoccupation with fitness: classes oftentimes are grueling and highly athletic. I often have students ask me if yoga is a good "workout." I am shocked when I discover that many people have been instructed in yoga without any mention of the breath at all. Deep breathing practice, after all, is a key to receiving the most nourishing and transformative aspect of energy (what yogis call *prana*) that life has to offer, and provides a panacea to facial aging. When I teach in gyms, I feel the need to explain the origins of yoga and its purpose to my students. Yoga was originally developed by monastics who spent hours at a time in meditation. They found that they needed to counter the cramps, gas, and stiffness caused by long periods of sitting. And so they began to develop the asanas, or poses. The name for yoga itself (from the Sanskrit word *yuj*, meaning to yoke or join together) really describes the yogic state of wholeness and integration. Today many of us modern Westerners sit for long periods, too, if not in contemplation, then at least in protracted periods of concentration in front of a computer screen. This is why we have taken to asana and its benefits. But we are still obsessed with moving and busyness, and our faces reflect this stress.

We want so much to be good, to be loved, to be approved of, that we are willing to get on a treadmill of frantic pace and effort and stay on it until we drop. It's as though we have come to believe that life itself is a competitive sport. Quite simply, we are exhausted! It's no wonder we struggle with the same ten pounds, medicating with alcohol and food, distracting with consumption and entertainment, and then wonder why, after working so hard to attain the perfect bodies, our faces start to look like pinched prunes. Somehow we forgot our faces! And by the time we notice, the damage seems to be irrevocable.

The Anatomy of the Face

When I was trained in drama school, on the first day of class my theatrical makeup professor told us to go home and "get to know" our faces. We were encouraged to liberally touch our faces until we knew them intimately: each plane, contour, pocket, and fleshy fold. Being in our twenties, most of us didn't find too many sags or wrinkles.

The most mesmerizing and illuminating exercise came toward the end of the class: the old-age makeup. We were told to pucker up and scrunch our features, and wherever lines emerged, we were to paint on those lines directly with our dark tint–dipped makeup brushes. It was fascinating to map out the future ravages of time. I can remember being genuinely humbled at the sight of what I would look like as a senior citizen. I looked angrier and more worried with my age lines. Actually, I looked like a person I might want to avoid in the street!

I learned from my makeup professor that as people age, their character becomes more defined. This is expressed through how we dress, walk, eat, and so on, but nowhere is character more clearly expressed as we age than *on the face*. People who have been happy and peaceful tend to have lines that go up rather than down because they have smiled more than they have frowned. People who worry will unconsciously play this emotion out on their faces over and over through repetitive puckering of the brow or clamping of the jaw and lips until the telltale line between the eyebrows turns into a furrowed and irrevocable crease and the line between the lips and nose (the nasal labial fold) deepens into a permanent frown. I have been a worrier, so my default expression is often a furrowed brow. This line was already showing up on my face through unconscious muscular repetition that day in class, but I had to scrunch and exaggerate it to see it in its early stages.

We also learned in makeup class that aging was primarily a process of dragging down: the laws of gravity would go into effect, and everything would start falling and drooping. Unfortunately, the hubris of youth told me it wasn't something I really needed to worry about it. I could wash the old-age makeup off, after all. I caught a glimpse of the future and pretty much ignored it. If only I had heeded the signs earlier. But then I might have not written this book.

Facial aging is a process of the facial features dragging down and sagging. But it is not just gravity that creates this syndrome. The skin contains a protein fiber called collagen, which in conjunction with another protein called elastin, is responsible for keeping the skin plump and firm. As we age, our skin slows down the production of collagen, and the firmness of the skin begins to go. When elastin stops being produced, we lose springiness and resilience, and that's when visible facial aging really begins. Test this out for yourself: lightly grip some facial skin between your thumb and index finger and give a little tug, then let go. Watch your skin resume its shape, and observe its resilience. This is your collagen and elastin working.

Skin is a highly sophisticated organ, covering our bodies in a protective sheath, sensing stimuli from the outside world, and informing us of vital information such as temperature. Skin serves as a temperature regulator, or thermostat, keeping our internal bodies at a functional level of warmth. Skin is also the body's detoxifier—through the sweat glands, it sloughs off the body's waste and external debris. Skin is composed of a few different layers, and contains sebaceous glands that produce sebum (a lubricant that coats and protects the skin), fatty cells, muscles, nerves, hair follicles, and hair.

The structure of the face is like the rest of the body. Skin covers layers of fat, muscle, connective tissue, and bone. Skin acts as a protective layer, and holds in its contents. The bone is the structural foundation, and the muscles are responsible for movement and protection of bone. When muscles are sedentary or largely inactive, fat develops to fill in a protective layer between the bone and skin, so that is why we must develop and train our facial muscles.

The muscles of the face, like the rest of the body, are subdivided into two categories: voluntary and involuntary. Larger muscles tend to be voluntary, and we tell them to help us do everything, from sitting to standing to running. But since the facial muscles are smaller and are not used to propel us forward or grasp anything, much of their movement is involuntary and uniquely expressive of emotion. But we can train our muscles through mental command and practice so that involuntary muscles can act voluntarily.

We are all aware of the positive benefits of exercise. But exercise should not stop at the neckline. The facial muscles deserve to be toned and firm as the crowning glory to a well-developed below-the-neck anatomy. Why on earth ignore your face? I believe that we haven't truly meant to neglect our facial muscles; we just don't know how to exercise them to obtain the results we'd like to see. That's why I created this book. In my research, I have come across many different facial exercises from many corners of the globe. People in countries from Hungary to Mongolia to India all practice some form of facial exercise. Whatever your background, I suspect you have an aunt or grandmother who can show you her favorite chin-firming technique.

Facial muscles can benefit from exercise as much as any other muscles. But in order to tone them, we must learn to train them, and then we must practice. You don't go for a run once. You start with a mile, then a mile and a half, and so on, until perhaps one day you can run a brisk 5K race. It is a continuous process of building muscle memory through repetition and discipline.

With the facial training of the Yoga Face program, the exercise pays off quickly: the facial muscles are trained to help lift the skin, and drooping and sagging areas are lifted and firmed, minimizing and softening lines and wrinkles. In turn, the full-body yoga poses draw more freshly oxygenated blood to the face, giving your skin a rosiness and luminescence, and eliminating bloat, toxins, and dullness. The poses also stimulate and regulate hormonal function, which helps to prolong youth and counter aging. Yogic twists wring out toxins from the internal organs, and help the brain to receive signals more efficiently from the spinal cord, the information superhighway of the body and mind. Detoxification and improved nerve communication both contribute to de-aging the body, mind, and face.

You *can* counter the visible effects of aging through facial exercise, diet, and yogic techniques, the main components of the Yoga Face program. What's more, you can do it naturally, creatively, and with almost no expense. It's time to claim your glowing, ageless beauty. Let your radiant inner light shine through a toned and lustrous face.

The Yoga Face has had remarkable rejuvenative effects on the faces of my students. Here are some amazing examples:

Jack, an investment banker, came to me hobbled and stiff from a punishing regimen with his trainer. His work demanded that he travel and eat out in restaurants a lot, and as a result he battled extra weight around the waistline and incredible stiffness. His attitude seemed to be the classic type-A "No pain, no gain"—if it didn't hurt, it didn't count. Then he'd "reward" himself at the end of a twelve-hour day with excessive wine-drinking with clients, still on the clock, after all. Early the next morning, he'd "sweat it out" with his trainer, lifting and running. Through diligence and remarkable will, he had already lost forty pounds when I started working with him. But he could barely walk, much less bend easily. He suffered from back pain and carrying those "last twenty" extra pounds. His face was puffy and bloated, from sleep deprivation and poor diet. I had an inkling Jack was more than a little stressed out.

In the beginning, I sometimes had Jack stand in Tadasana (the basic standing pose) for five minutes at a time, while focusing on his alignment and breath. At first, this standing practice was a challenge, but it was all he could really manage. Sitting in a cross-legged position was impossible—his hips were too tight. Over time, standing became easier. Eventually he could sit cross-legged, and finally he could touch his toes as well. But when he simply practiced the standing pose, he began to breathe more easily. And with the breathing, his face transformed. The color returned, and eventually he lost that bloated quality. His skin got smoother. I turned him on to easy inversions, and his face dropped ten years in appearance. He began modifying his diet and exercise regimen, incorporating a less-is-more approach, and today he is transformed.

I noticed that as we began to do more restorative poses, Jack's face got lighter and smoother. I began applying some acupressure techniques to his face in the resting poses, and I marveled as his face lost some of the flabbiness and excess weight. The contours of his face—particularly in the jaw and cheek area—reemerged with more definition, and his face gave a more youthful appearance.

Marcia is a fit and fabulous surgical nurse. She has taken care of herself, and it shows. Though in her early fifties, she could easily pass for a vibrant forty-something. She started attending my classes about a year ago, and she has gotten more radiant, dewy, and supple than ever. Because of her medical background, Marcia knew that the Yoga Face program was scientifically grounded and made good sense. She tells me she's been sharing the Yoga Face exercises with some of her patients. Recently she's been working as an on-set nurse in the movie industry, and she has been giving the Yoga Face tips to the actresses and makeup crew. She especially likes the Marilyn exercise (see page 16), and swears it has plumped her lips noticeably.

Rianna is a beautiful, creative woman who took to my class right away. A forty-something writer and designer, she has been concerned about her biological clock, and the physiological changes she's been experiencing as she gets to the latter end of her child-bearing years. Like many women today, Rianna focused on her career and personal growth, only to discover she forgot to have a baby! Now she wants to have a child, but is without a significant other. Being extremely sensitive, I think that sometimes she is prone to depression. So the emotional release of the Yoga Face has been a boon for her. She loves the expressive portion of the class. The emotive aspect of releasing breath and the sound work really tickle her—in class she's prone to break out in spontaneous peals of laughter. Rianna has clearly benefited from the emotional release that the Yoga Face provides. Her energy is infectious, and her demeanor has shifted from sullen to glowing. In addition, the worry and frown lines that used to give the appearance of a permanent scowl have eased, and she looks noticeably more youthful as a result.

Then there's Roberta, a beauty industry professional who's always looked great. I have seen major transformation in the year she's been my student. Roberta is fit and attractive, but the droopy bags around her eyes were getting her down. I gave her a few simple inversions such as to practice Legs-Up-the-Wall (page 71) and Downward-Facing Dog (page 72), and the results have been fantastic: she has lost the bagginess around her eyes. And with a few of the eye-lift exercises, she has countered the downward creases around her eyes and reduced her crow's-feet. She looks great, and it shows—she's gotten engaged since she started my program!

Jan and Doug came to me three years ago. When I first met them, I was struck by their physical fitness: they both worked out with a personal trainer, and although they were in their early fifties, they had the physiques of people twenty years younger. But they both were concerned with maintaining their attractive youthfulness, and they were getting Restylane and botox injections. One day, Jan could barely move her mouth as a result of collagen injections. She had bruises on her face, and consequently had to cancel a social engagement for later that evening. When I saw her a day or two later, the swelling had gone down and the bruises had diminished, but her range of facial expression was still restricted. My hunch was that Jan could find alternatives to distressing and lifting her face. Through developing a consistent yoga practice with me and adjusting her diet, Jan's facial appearance began to change. I am happy to report that it's been two years since Jan has felt the need to have any facial procedures, and she looks more unlined now than she did then. Her skin is more firm and less hollowed-out-looking, and it totally glows.

Doug has also greatly benefited from this system. After practicing the relaxation and breathing techniques, he has dropped a perpetual involuntary scowl along with the lines around his mouth, eyes, and forehead that used to accompany it. In addition, a steady inversion practice of Headstand (page 73) and Shoulderstand (page 69) have stimulated his hormonal production, and given him increased virility and a thicker head of hair.

Maude, in her early fifties, is an athletic and attractive woman. But her face was beginning to show some signs of aging: her lips were thinning, and the lines around them were deepening. Additionally, she had a pucker line between her brows that made her look older than she felt. I selected two target-area facial exercises (Marilyn, page 16, and Surprise Me!, page 33) and recommended that she practice cooling inversions such as Shoulderstand (page 69) or Legs-Up-the-Wall Pose (page 71). She has lost the lines around her mouth and between her eyes, and the inversions have helped her to stay more rosy and relaxed looking.

Dr. Bainbridge, a seventy-something public official, came to me because of lower back pain. His constant overbooking and "bending over backward" to help others left him chronically stiff and hunched over—the physical manifestations of carrying the weight of the world on his shoulders. His long and successful career had been built on helping everyone else and neglecting himself, and he had a lot of back pain to show for it. This stress also manifested itself as a cramped neck and an involuntary facial grimace of tension. This was his physical response to a busy life in public service. Once we started working together, I saw that he needed to slow down and *receive* energy rather than only give it away as he so generously does in his daily life. I gave him restorative poses that would lightly stimulate hormonal function (such as Fish Pose, page 75), and taught him some meditation and breathing techniques to help regulate his heart rate and receive more oxygen, and was pleased to see that his face really relaxed, got smoother, and became more radiant after each session.

All of these clients, though quite different in age and profession, shared a common underlying problem: they all wanted to feel better and look younger, but didn't realize that they could actually accomplish this by slowing down, and intelligently going to the source of their stress and facial aging. The facial exercises, calming techniques, and emotional release that I shared with them helped them de-age visibly, quickly, and easily. And they got the added benefit of relaxation.

My hope is that through *The Yoga Face* you will find a fun and creative way to counter the effects of aging in your facial appearance, and, even more, that you may find a truly rejuvenating way of life that is more than just skin deep. In this book, I will give you some wonderful techniques for facial rejuvenation. I encourage you to play with these methods and gauge the results not only on your face but also in your life. You may just find both your skin and your outlook transformed.

chapter two

The Facial Exercises

Your face is your emotional canvas. It is your brand: the label, or logo, by which others identify who you are. Like it or not, your face carries all your thoughts, feelings, and impressions, and then transmits them to the world instantaneously. The face also acts as an archive, or record bank, of your emotions, which is why the more one ages, the more one's character is revealed. You may be in the habit of scrunching your brow in response to life's frustrations, which will in time show up as a pinched line between the brows. Or you may have a habitual tendency to "swallow rage," rather than express your feelings, which may manifest in your jaw's becoming clenched and your shoulders hunched. Similarly, fear can cause the corners of the mouth to downturn in a grimacing frown. Whatever your predominant emotions, they will be reflected in your facial appearance.

As an experiment, observe other people's faces in public, perhaps when you are on the train to work or dining in a restaurant. Most telling are the faces that are alone in silent reverie—the unguarded expressions of strangers who don't know they are being observed speak volumes. When people forget they are in public, all sorts of interesting facial habits can be witnessed. I am always shocked at the sad, angry, or lonely expressions I see in the faces of those around me. Little scowls, twitches from tension, puckered lips, and furrowed brows are all evidence of the myriad emotions that play out on our faces unbeknown to ourselves. Even if a person is not upset, concentration can cause all kinds of puckers and frowns on the face, which when repeated over and over will start to show up as permanent expressions in the form of wrinkles. But don't despair! You *do* have control over what your face transmits. Contrary to what many think, the face is not a static mask, nor is it—in its present condition—something you are stuck with. With conscious practice and exercise, the face is quite malleable. Plastic surgeons have often referred to the sculptural quality of their work, and are quite right in regarding the face as raw material.

You *can* change your face. As I mentioned earlier, sometimes I used to catch myself off guard when I would see my reflection in a shop window—and I'd crack up at the silly scowl contorting my face. Now I have trained myself to maintain a neutral expression with a small smile of contentment as I walk through my daily tasks. If I do catch my reflection in a window, it tends to be more serene, and my facial appearance has smoothed considerably through this easy yet effective form of muscular training. And because I look pleasantly relaxed, I find that people treat me more congenially and life flows more easily. Doors open, both literally and metaphorically!

Through the practice of the Yoga Face, you can positively transform your face without any surgery at all. Think of this as a creative act: have fun with the process, and get ready to create a masterpiece on the canvas of your skin. Gently guiding your facial muscles through daily reminders to smile or at least be neutral rather than puckering, frowning, or scowling will go a long way in erasing or easing emotional patterns that have become part of your facial expression. And there is a very active tool you can use as well: facial exercise!

The following exercises are facial isolations that can be used as a sequence. Or you may pick and choose the ones you think are best for your face. For instance, if you have begun to notice signs of wrinkles in your brows or forehead, refer to the brow and forehead exercises in this chapter. If you are concerned about keeping your lips firm and full, use the Marilyn exercise on a daily basis. If it's your throat or jaw area that seems in need of firming and sculpting, use the Baby Bird or another exercise from the cluster that deals with this area. Each exercise cluster deals with a different part of the face, though if you want to keep your face in the best possible condition, I suggest you do all of these exercises daily. Once you achieve mastery of them, they won't take more than six to eight minutes in total to practice. Do these exercises after a face cleansing, when you have applied some light moisturizer and the skin is a little slick. Morning or evening is fine—whichever you prefer. Think of these exercises as the scales a musician practices daily to stay in shape—only with you, your expressive in-strument is your face and its muscles. You will notice that as you practice these "scales" more frequently, your facial agility will improve, and your range of expression will im-prove with your increased "face-ility." While the exercises are effective because they engage the facial muscles, they also facilitate emotional release. Thus, letting go of tension and worry in the face is also an instant rejuvenator.

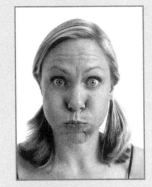

1. Satchmo

This exercise is named after the inimitable Louis Armstrong. If you observe photographs of his cheeks, or any other trumpet player's cheeks, you will see that they are firm and strong, long into old age. Years of engaging these muscles keeps them resilient. The muscles used to blow are the buccinators (they are the "apples" that form when you smile, lifting your cheeks up). If you exercise yours, they will stay strong and supple as well. Recall the joyful exuberance of Satchmo's face as he played his horn, and use that ebullience as you firm your cheeks.

Mechanics:

Puff up both cheeks with air, then transfer air from cheek to cheek. Alternate back and forth until you are out of breath. Repeat three or four times.

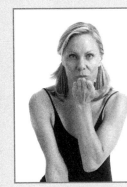 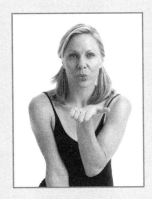

2. Marilyn

This exercise will strengthen the ring muscles around the mouth and create stronger, firmer lips. It is also a mood elevator. As you blow glamorous kisses, visualize throngs of admiring fans.

Mechanics:

While keeping your brow smooth and unruffled, isolate your facial muscles to blow kisses. Repeat three or four times.

Now add resistance by pressing your lips to your first two fingers. Pucker your lips and press lightly into the fingertips. Do three or four repetitions.

3. Sphinx Smile

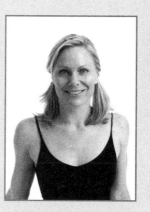

Now is the time to examine your smile. Smiling and laughing invariably create grooves in the skin through their constant repetition, but if you observe your smile in the mirror, you can eradicate tendencies to inadvertently groove unnecessary lines into the face.

Mechanics:

Smile by lifting the corners of your mouth up and across, but keep your eyes neutral. Keep relaxed and smooth as you smile. Imagine you possess a mysterious secret—perhaps the answer to a long unsolved riddle! Do this three or four times, and ingrain the feeling of this smile into your muscle memory.

4. Tongue Tracing

This exercise will help keep your lips plump and your cheeks firm. It tones the neck and throat as well. It will also facilitate jaw release.

Mechanics:

Open your mouth in a perfect "O" shape. Trace your tongue around the entire circumference of your lips, first one direction, and then in the opposite direction. Keep your lower jaw relaxed, and your forehead and brows smooth. Repeat three or four times.

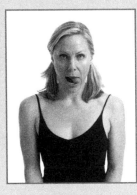 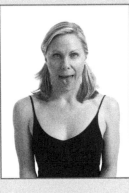

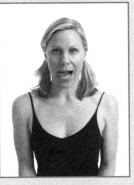 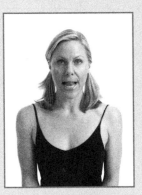

5. Smiling Fish Face

At some point, celebrities must have examined their faces and made a conscious decision to combine a smile with a pout (a "smout") for the camera. Probably they did this consciously to mold their faces for the paparazzi, knowing the photos were being transmitted to millions of viewers. This exercise will help firm and tone your cheeks and lips, so that you, too, will be ready for the paparazzi!

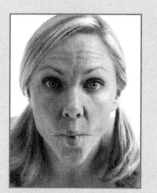

Mechanics:

Smile while slightly pursing your lips. Withdraw and pinch your cheeks into the hollows of your face slightly as you do so, observing the enhanced cheekbones this pose creates. Repeat four to five times, or for a total of ten to fifteen seconds.

I do not recommend habitually posing like this, as it is rather affected, but it is a good exercise for the mirror, and it will work the ring muscles of the mouth as well as the buccinators.

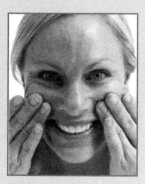

6. Puppet Face

This exercise smooths and lifts marionette lines, the lines between the nose and lips. It works the muscles that lift the lips up in a smile, preventing and smoothing jowls.

Mechanics:

Smile and press your fingertips into the crease that forms between the lips and nose. Perform repetitions by lifting these muscles up in a smiling action, while pressing the fingertips down on the area for resistance. Repeat twenty to thirty times. Notice the increased circulation manifesting as rosiness in the area when you have finished.

7. Free Your Tongue and Your Throat Will Follow

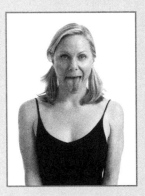

The tongue is the only muscle we can take out of our body at will. It needs stretching and toning like all muscles. As you perform this exercise, be mindful of the tingling—the burn—of working out this important muscle.

Mechanics:

Stick out your tongue and say *aaaaah*, then hold it out while keeping the rest of your face relaxed for sixty seconds. Your eyes may water. (That's good—it will flush out any toxins you may have accumulated there.) Sixty seconds is a long time, isn't it?

8. Kiss the Ceiling

This is a great jaw, neck, and throat firmer. It also helps plump the lips and keep them firm and full.

Mechanics:

Standing, tilt your head slightly back and try to "kiss the ceiling." Stretch the lips and pucker up. Repeat this four times.

The lower jaw is the only bone in the head that can move independently of the skull, because it is hinged to the upper jaw. This mobility is partially because the ligaments and muscles of the jaw are powerful enough to pull an automobile, or, in Jack La Lanne's case, a small tugboat. In addition to chewing, we use the jaw for speech and expression. Jaw tension can cause a lot of unpleasant symptoms: TMJ, a condition in which chronic grinding of the teeth can lead to headaches, loss of tooth enamel, wearing down of the teeth, which can cause nerve exposure, and, by extension, root canals and nerve pain, and unattractive facial wrinkling around the mouth, lips, and nasal-labial area. Luckily, there are many ways to free tension from the jaw, and in doing so release the facial muscles from uncomfortable and unattractive clenching and tightness. Relaxing the jaw through the following exercises will help your face to look much smoother and more youthful. Some of these exercises involve sound, which travels in waves, and vibration, which can subtly release tension as well.

It is important to note that it is imperative to leave the rest of the face and head as relaxed as possible when working with jaw-releasing techniques that involve vocalization. Don't jut out your neck as you perform the exercises. Keep releasing your lower jaw and the back of the throat and palate as well.

1. Warm-up: Slack Jaw

Involuntarily gripping the jaw is an indication of frustration and tension. It can also signal a type-A tendency to want to be perfect, to hold it all in, to control. Think of the classic military face of General Patton as portrayed by George C. Scott. Also, when sadness and grief are repressed, the jaw clenches as though to swallow the emotion.

Mechanics:

For this exercise, give yourself permission to let it all hang out—literally. Release your lower jaw from the upper so that your teeth are parted. You can let the tip of the tongue rest behind your lower teeth. Let your head be centered on top of your spine. Let your eyes relax in their sockets, and relax your face. Consider this the neutral posture that you can start your jaw-releasing work from. Place your fingertips on your lower jaw to facilitate this release.

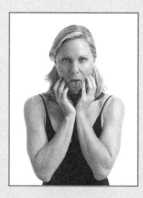

2. Bumblebees

This exercise helps work the cheeks, lips, and jaw muscles, while simultaneously releasing jaw tension. It employs vibration as a method of disarming tension. Pay attention to the vibratory quality of the sound as you chew, and notice how the vibration produces a fuzzy tingle as it resonates and bounces off the bones of the jaw and cheeks. As you become more adept, start to play with vibrating sound from all areas of the head—even try to vibrate your scalp and the base of the skull. Place a hand on the area you are working.

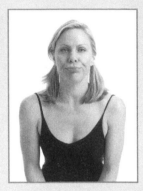

Mechanics:

Inhale through your nose and begin to make a chewing sound. Use all the muscles of the face. Vibrate the sound *mmmmm* through your nose as you exhale and chew. Repeat for three or four full breaths. Experiment with different pitches, perhaps high, then low. Then re-peat the exercise, but this time incorporate gibberish words. Using the word *why* as you chew can be especially cathartic, as it allows you to release any self-pity or dramatic feelings you sometimes may need to repress. Go ahead, emote and express, be dramatic—you prob-ably will crack yourself up!

3. Open Wide and Say Aaaaah

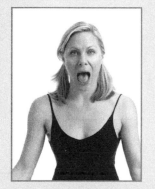

You probably have released quite a bit of tension, and you should see instant results. Gripping in the jaw is often a sign of unexpressed emotion—particularly the taboo emotions of anger and grief. If you have ever felt like bursting into tears or giving someone a piece of your mind, but instead had to hold your tongue or swallow your words, chances are those unexpressed emotions are literally lodged in your jaw.

At the more extreme end of this syndrome are those who clench habitually or grind their teeth at night. Those who experience this level of jaw tension will enjoy considerable release from the jaw-releasing work employed here. Having suffered from a lot of jaw tension during my performing career, and also being a nocturnal jaw grinder, I cannot recommend highly enough the tooth guard my dentist prescribed for me. I sleep much better and awaken more refreshed. Also, consider letting go of chewing gum, as it adds to jaw tension and literally can help to set more tension in the face.

Mechanics:

Now vary the sound so that it is *mmmmmmm-aaaaah mmmmmmm-aaaaah mmmmmmmm-aaaaah*. As you alternate between humming *mmmmmm* through the nose and opening the mouth to say *aaaaah*, notice the variations of the sound vibrations. When you say *aaaaah*, let your lower jaw release, and tuck the tip of your tongue behind the lower teeth. This will allow your jaw to release even more, and sound will come out with less inhibition.

This exercise cycle is a mega-release and should be practiced as much as possible. Notice how your face looks after several minutes.

4. Heart Chakra Opener

Producing the sound *aaaaah* will also create vibration in the chest center. Perhaps it is for this reason that the *aaaaah* sound is considered to be a heart chakra opener. You may experiment with this further by taking Easy Pose (Sukhasana) and chanting the *aaaaah* sound while placing your left hand on your crown center at the top of the skull and your right hand at the center of your chest. Make sure your mouth is wide open and that your tongue is low and relaxed in your mouth to get the maximum jaw release and best quality of sound. Chant *aaaaah* and rub your hands to coax the vibration out more fully. Try this two to four times, then close your eyes and experience the warm and radiant quality of an open heart. An open heart will instantly transform the face from a shut-down, pinched mask to an open, radiant, and glowing goddess face.

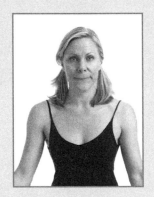

5. Baby Bird

This exercise will assist in firming the chin, neck, and cheeks. It helps prevent jowls from forming and is a good antidote for existing ones.

Mechanics:

Tilt your head back and look at the ceiling. You must be relaxed when doing this—it is a bit challenging at first. Swallow while pressing the tip of your tongue to the roof of your mouth. Then tilt your head slightly to the left and swallow. Tilt your head slightly to the right and swallow. Do three to four times in each direction.

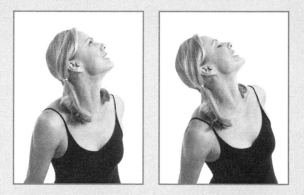

6. Head and Neck Rolls

The tension this exercise releases will illuminate your face by lifting pinched or glum expressions, and it will also tone the neck, throat, and chin.

Releasing head and neck tension serves to "prime the canvas" of facial release. Once you have loosened up this area, you will find your head sits more easily upon your shoulders and your posture improves. Improved posture helps the entire body, as the spine is freed from constriction and the abdominal muscles are properly engaged to support the spine, translating into a slimmer, more sculpted physical profile. You will also create a new sense of lightness that releases the sense of burden that a tight neck and shoulders produce. Your face will automatically release and look less pinched and constricted, ultimately resulting in fewer wrinkles.

Mechanics:

Keep your head squarely perched on top of your neck, and imagine a silver thread connected to the crown of your head on one end, and to a point at the top of the sky on the other. Imagine the thread lengthening and lifting your entire spine.

Now gently roll your head from shoulder to shoulder, leading with the chin. Make the motions small and precise. Then explore small circular motions—by performing full head rolls—but if this bothers your neck, stay with half-circular motions instead.

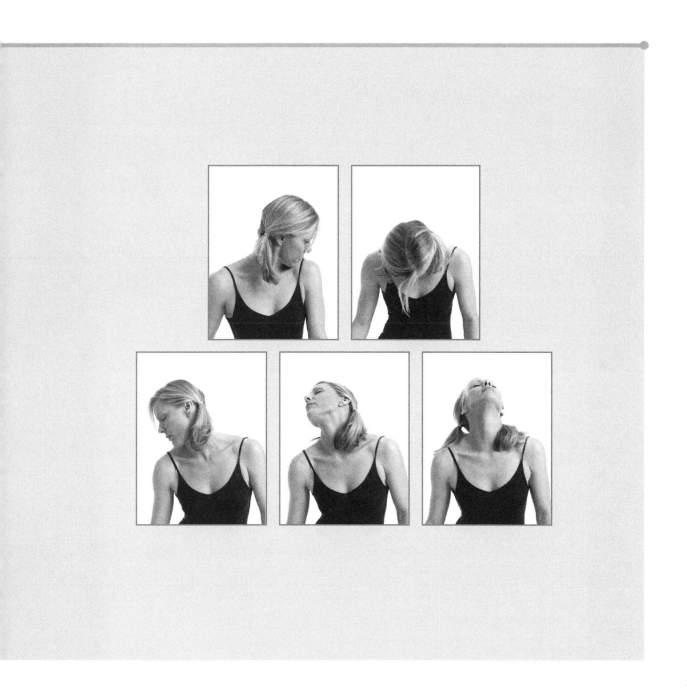

7. The Lower Jaw Grip and Shake

This exercise is a mega-release, and will help anyone who suffers from pucker lines around the lips—when it looks like you're sucking a lemon, permanently—as well as worry lines between the eyebrows and above the brows. Releasing the jaw also unburdens "trapped" emotions of anger, repressed desire, and sadness that tend to lodge in this area.

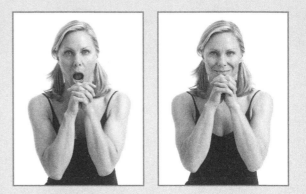

Mechanics:

Interlace your fingers (but not the thumbs). Tuck your thumbs under your lower jaw, in the indentation behind the lower jaw ridge. Place your interlaced fingers (index fingers on top) under your lips, on the chin, like you are lightly grabbing a handle. Let your lower jaw loosen and drop down, becoming slack. Lightly gripping your lower jaw, move your interlaced fingers up and down, saying *aaaaah* as you go. This is a huge jaw release and may be a gauge of how tense you are. If you find it almost impossible to isolate the lower jaw's movement from the upper jaw's, you have a lot of jaw tension, and this exercise is for you! The jaw is a hinge, so let the other exercises be a lubricant that starts working the jaw. Even if it feels daunting now, with practice, you will be able to perform this more advanced exercise. Remember, easy does it! Practice this three to four times in a row, for about two minutes or so.

8. Sandbag

This exercise stretches the neck, shoulders, and jaw, and will let your head sit more effortlessly on your neck, reducing the appearance of jowls or double chins, and preventing them from forming through the practice of good posture.

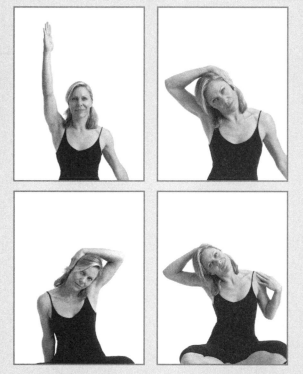

Mechanics:

In a seated pose, walk the fingertips of your left hand along the floor ten inches or so to the left of your hip. Rest lightly on your left fingertips. Extend your right arm up with your palm rotated in toward your right cheek. Then bend your arm at the right elbow and clasp your left ear with your right palm. Keeping your head aligned on your neck, drop your head toward the right and apply a gentle pressure, or sandbag, to the left ear. If you want to go deeper with this stretch, take your left fingertips (palm-down) to your left upper arm and apply a little pressure. Hold for five to seven counts, perhaps increasing the sandbag weight, then repeat on the other side.

Exercise Cluster: Forehead and Eyes

The eyes may be the windows of the soul, but unfortunately they can be obscured by heavy drapes of bags and wrinkles. And sometimes the sills need a little renovation. This area tends to be the most glaring (forgive the pun) indicator of damage and neglect. But do not despair. You can restore a youthful look to the delicate skin around the eyes through exercise.

1. *Temple Dancer Eyes*

Kathak dancers in India perform eye movements with as much elegance and precision as ballerinas performing *rondes des jambes*. These eye movements exercise the ring muscles of the eyes, healing and preventing sagging skin and crow's-feet.

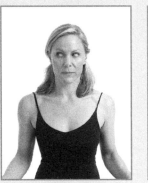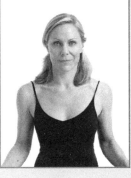
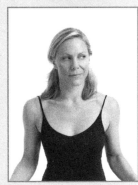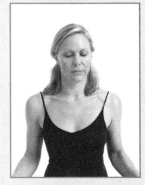

Mechanics:

With your head held erect at the top of your spine, move your eyes to look to the left, then center, then right. Do not move your face or neck. Simply dart your eyes from side to center to side, then reverse the direction. Do not hold your gaze for any length of time. Repeat three times. Then close your eyes and "look down" toward your nose.

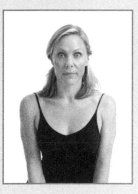

2. Surprise Me!

This is a major brow smoother and de-wrinkler. It also exercises the ring muscles around the eyes, firming and lifting the eye area. Because the frontalis muscle is employed (a very large facial muscle connected to the scalp) it is relatively easy to do, and can be mastered quickly. Look for the rosy glow in the forehead and brow region after you do this exercise—it is proof that circulation is traveling to the target area.

Mechanics:

Widen your eyes as though you are very surprised, being careful to not wrinkle the brow. Focus on a point at the horizon line (it can be imaginary) for about five to ten seconds. Repeat four times.

3. Buddha Face

This is a relaxation exercise to help neutralize tension and release unconscious clenching, tightening, and furrowing that lead to wrinkles. You can practice this while riding the subway, in your car, or in the doctor's waiting room. The more you can practice this on a regular basis, the smoother your face will be.

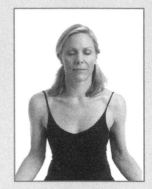

When all is said and done, nothing works better than a calm countenance for cultivating a serene inner disposition. The face is the transmitter of emotion, and you can manipulate it to change yourself from the outside in. In other words, you can design your inner state by picking a face that will facilitate the mood. Imagine that your face is a beautiful accessory, a crowning jewel that completes your look. Before you go out for your day, do this exercise and choose the ultimate accessory—facial serenity.

Mechanics:

You can do this exercise either in a standing position after you have completed the other facial exercises, or in a seated posture. Close your eyes and concentrate on consciously smoothing out all wrinkles. Imagine a point between the brows—a small iridescent disc of light—and with your mind's eye, watch it expand. If you feel your mind drift off, bring your attention back to the point between the brows, mentally smoothing the facial muscles as you do so. Start with one minute, then work up to two or three. In a seated posture, you may do this for as long as you like.

4. Crow, Crow, Go Away!

This exercise works to prevent or reverse drooping and sagging in the lower lids of the eyes, and also to uncrease crow's-feet.

Mechanics:

Start by smiling. Next, place your index finger on the crease. Now pulse your lower eyelid muscles against the resistance of the index finger's pressure. This is an isolation movement, so do not move any other facial muscles. Do twenty repetitions. After you become adept, try forty.

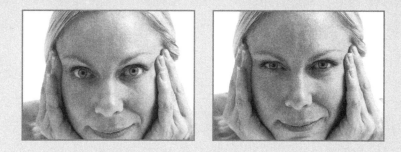

5. Brow Lift

This exercise firms the frontalis muscle, the largest muscle on the forehead, which connects to the skull. Exercising this muscle is easier than exercising some of the smaller facial muscles.

Mechanics:

Raise the muscle above the eyebrows (you will see folds as you lift here). Now take one fingertip of each hand and smooth the creases above the outer eyebrow out toward the temple, while clasping your palms to the temples.

Raise the frontalis muscles against the resistance of the fingertip pressure. Keep the other facial muscles as neutral as possible. Lift and release the frontalis as rapidly as you can, while applying fingertip pressure, for a cycle of twenty. Repeat once. Observe the rosy glow in your skin after completing this exercise—circulation is traveling to the area.

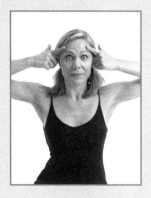

1. Lion Face (Simhasana)

This is a classic yoga pose for the face that stretches all the facial muscles and releases emotional tension. Do not be afraid to really tighten and constrict your facial muscles, for you will follow the constriction with a big release. Imagine a situation or a person that is frustrating you as you contract the face. You will feel a beneficial flush of circulation after the release of the constriction. Note the rosy glow in your skin after you've completed the exercise.

Mechanics:

Inhale through your nose, make fists, and squeeze all the facial muscles as if you have sucked a very tart lemon. Then simultaneously exhale through your mouth, stick out your tongue, roll your eyes up, and open your hands. Repeat three times.

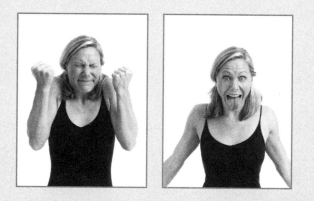

2. Tongue Twisters

After releasing the lips, jaw, and cheeks in the previous exercise, notice how much more command you have in speaking. You can play with this new ease by repeating tongue twisters. They are fun to do, and will also help keep your facial muscles supple. Try each one about five times. Do not jut the neck or tense the face! Increase the tempo as you become more adept.

1. "What a to-do to die today at a minute or two to two. A distinctly difficult thing to say, but harder still to do. For they'll beat a tattoo at a twenty to two with a rat-a-ta-tat-ta-ta-tat-ta-ta-too, and the dragon will come when he hears the drum at a minute or two to two today, at a minute or two to two."
2. "You know New York, you need New York, you know you need unique New York."
3. "Red leather, yellow leather, good blood, bad blood."

These exercises are the cornerstone of facial fitness. When steadily practiced, you will notice a difference in your face, as it looks firmer, smoother, and more relaxed. The added benefits of jaw tension release and a sunnier, more serene disposition will contribute to a refreshed appearance. The freedom from neck and shoulder tension these simple exercises afford will also improve your shoulder, neck, and head posture, aiding in the prevention of unattractive jowls and double chins. You can relax, knowing that you have a program to keep your face radiant, firm, and supple.

chapter three

Traditional Yoga Poses That Help the Face

When I first started practicing yoga, my face began to transform. I wasn't exactly sure how, but I started looking younger. The yoga teachers and enthusiasts I polled acknowledged that their faces were changing, but none could explain why. They seemed to assume that a smoother, more youthful face was a mysterious benefit of yoga, certainly a gift horse not to be looked in the mouth. But once I started realizing I was obtaining facial benefits from the poses, I wanted more—and as soon as possible! I began to devise a system to categorize poses by their facially rejuvenating qualities. I researched and practiced, then took my findings to my students and watched them transform rapidly.

Facial aging is not caused by one particular culprit, but is rather a combination of different factors. Similarly, the visible signs of aging manifest differently, and in differing ratios, depending on the patterns and habits of the individual. These are the main effects of facial aging:

Loss of tone: As we age, we lose collagen and elastin, the proteins that combine to form resilience and to firm the skin. This loss creates a general drooping or sagginess.

Wrinkles: Wrinkles are formed by losing elasticity, and also by the tension that causes unconscious facial clenching and grimacing, setting the facial muscles in habitual expressions that, over time, create a perma-expression, or mask.

Color: Poor circulation, toxins, and accumulated dead skin on the skin's surface affect its color, creating a dull, ashy, or grayish quality. Accumulated toxins in the system show up as age spots and discolorations on the skin.

Dry skin: Excess toxins dry out the skin (think of the dehydrating properties of caffeine, alcohol, and sugar) and deplete the skin's cells of oxygen. Toxins can also backlog in the skin to create puffiness and bloat. Whether the skin becomes drier and more papery, or puffier and less defined, these hydration issues are really two sides of the same coin.

These four major signifiers of facial aging have four corresponding yogic antidotes. They are grouped into category by color and corresponding element. The color/element categories assigned to the poses in this chapter are to help you choose which exercises are best for you, but in fact all yoga poses address aspects of each element. In selecting poses for facial anti-aging, choose a pose that addresses your problem area, but also be open to trying poses that may not be on your radar. Some facial aging happens beneath the surface, undetected. Most of the problems I address here are universal, so it is best to prevent problems before they start.

The *bandhas* are energy locks that are applied to different points on the body in asana and breathing practice. Although the bandhas are physical, they are used to direct the subtle energy pathways as well as the physical body. There are two major energy pathways, one that flows up and one that flows down. It is thought that when we become imbalanced, redirecting downward-flowing energy upward and vice versa will cause revitalization and balance. From a physical standpoint, employing the bandhas energizes and strengthens the practice, and enhances its benefits. Since redirecting downward-flowing energy results in bringing life force, or *prana*, back up, this directly benefits the face by imparting much-needed circulation, color, and vigor back up to the chest, lungs, and face. You can see the effects in improved color and tone. Also, the cells are able to revitalize more efficiently.

The three major bandhas I will describe in application to the exercises in this book are:

Mulabandha, or root lock. This lock will be applied by gathering in the pelvic floor area between the anus and the genitals (the perineum), and applying a subtle lift in the vaginal muscles if you are a woman. You can also think of applying this lock as "drawing in the sit bones" toward each other.

Uddiyana Bandha, or "flying up" lock. After an exhale, without taking in a new breath, draw up the area two inches below the navel, and keep this lock lightly drawing in to subvert downward-flowing energy, and to engage the abdominal core muscles. This lock is very effective in employing core strength, and especially in "gravity defying" poses that require balance, such as Handstand (page 68) and Crow (page 55). Also, this lock extends the spine and is a wonderful tool to deepen forward bending. Do not practice this lock when pregnant.

Jalandhara Bandha, or "capping off" or throat lock. Often used as the final lock after the other two have been implemented. Lift the sternum toward the chin, and drop the chin slightly toward the sternal notch. This is often practiced in conjunction with breath retention and will help to seal in and retain the prana that has been lifted from the lower body. After this lock has been released, you will see a rosy glow on your face and feel a renewed sense of energy and mental clarity. You may experience a little light-headedness while performing this lock.

A note on directions in asana practice:

In general, the right side of the body is considered to be masculine, and the left to be feminine. Therefore, practicing a pose for the first time on the right side is the traditional method. The thought behind this is that the right side is more fiery and aggressive, and the left is more receptive and cool, so practicing the pose first on the right will add heat and energy, and correspondingly dispel any excess energy. Practicing on the left side second will "cool down" and balance the physical as well as energetic body.

Another general rule, though by no means always true, is that whichever side is dominant tends to be stronger, and whichever side is less active will be more flexible. Most of us are right-handed; the left side tends to be more open and flexible and the right side stronger and more rigid. If you notice a great disparity between the two sides in your practice, you may wish to do more strengthening on your weak side by holding the pose a count or two longer, or increase flexibility on the rigid side by exhaling a count or two longer in a soothing pose (any of the forward bends). These patterns can be adjusted through conscientious observation and corresponding adjustments such as the ones I have suggested. Once you have corrected an imbalance, feel free to shift the adjustment you made to achieve balance.

A note on the times of poses:

In general, a pose should be held for five to eight breaths, counting the inhale and the exhale as one unit of breath. The major exception is Savasana, or Corpse Pose, where consciously noticing and/or counting breath is inappropriate as it is a resting pose. There is no mandate or exact time on suggested poses, as some will feel especially beneficial, and should be enjoyed and experienced as deeply as instinct dictates. That being said, balance is to be sought, and paying attention to the duration of poses will help the practioner to achieve equanimity in her practice. Paying attention to the breathing in poses will help to cultivate knowledge of one's tendencies and patterns. If you are unable to breathe deeply and easily in a pose, it may suggest that you have blocked energy, or resistance to what the pose has to offer. Or, it may be a cue that this pose is causing pain, in which case follow your breath's signal and make an adjustment in the pose or stop if you feel it isn't appropriate for you. Breathing deeply in poses increases the meditative aspects of each pose. It will also help you focus off the mat. Breathing in can be equated with an ability to experience and feel, whereas breathing out is associated with release, or letting go. Another way of regarding one's experience with breath is to think of the inhale as the effort, and the exhale as the grace. Ideally, these two should be in balance in terms of duration. If, however, one is prone to more effort and less comfortable with receiving grace, taking a little longer on an exhale as breathing exercise may be helpful.

Practice is an ongoing process of minor adjustments, and watchfulness in practice will help heal injuries and imbalances and prevent the onset of new ones. Remember that you are always the best judge of your tendencies. Listen to your intuition and inner voice as you practice and *never* ignore them.

Green/Earth: *The De-wrinklers*

Poses that draw upon the earth's regenerative qualities are especially good for tapping into earth energy (vitality) and life force. Applied to the face, this translates as rejuvenation. Earth corresponds to the first chakra, or energy center, and is therefore linked with the physical realm. The earth poses will help improve the overall vitality of the skin, hair, and teeth.

Targets: Smooths brow, de-wrinkles forehead, lifts eyes, and plumps and firms the mouth.

Blue/Water: *The Plumpers and Firmers*

The element of water is vital for keeping skin firm and full. Aging skin tends to shrivel and lose its dewiness—the poses in this category will help keep the face from losing its elasticity. Water's receptive nature ensures that it doesn't become rigid or stuck, so the water poses are also helpful for dissolving tension and clenching in the face. These poses also regulate excess water and will remove bloat and puffiness from the face. Water is replenishing and rejuvenating.

Targets: Counters dry skin, erases bags, fills hollows, plumps lips and cheeks. Alleviates puffiness, bloat, and loss of facial definition.

Silver/Air: *The Energizers*

Mercurial and quick, air is associated with prana, or life force. Using the poses in this category will help to redirect energy that is trapped below the neck and move it up to the face. These poses will help the lungs to receive and distribute more oxygen (most of us use only about a third of our lung capacity). This translates as increased circulation, and is therefore a major component in improving skin tone.

Targets: Improves circulation and, by extension, facial skin tone and skin color.

Red/Fire: *The Detoxifiers and Heaters*

Fire is used for burning away impurities. The heating properties of fire poses (or, in Sanskrit, *tapas*) act as detoxifiers. Since the skin is the body's largest excretory organ, it will benefit from having fewer impurities to process. These poses refresh and renew the face. They also improve circulation, which is helpful for cell regeneration.

Targets: Improves skin tone and counters sagginess, droopiness, and dull color. Turn up the heat in the body to bring increased vigor and energy.

To diagnose your problem areas, then match them with an appropriate exercise, look closely (but lovingly) at your face under a good strong light (avoid fluorescent light, as it makes your tone look off and yellow or greenish), first thing in the morning after your morning cleansing. To check your skin's tone and firmness, gently pull an area of skin between your index finger and thumb, then let go and watch how quickly it snaps back. Notice where the majority of the skin's loss of firmness is.

Some general guidelines when practicing all of these poses: relax your face, upturn the corners of your mouth in a neutral, sweet smile as you practice, and consciously relax your jaw. By parting your teeth a little and relaxing your tongue in these poses you will start to develop the good habit of keeping your face relaxed in the rest of your life. Make an *aaaaah* sound at the end of an exhale whenever you want to release facial tension. This will release your jaw muscles and facilitate facial relaxation.

I will give you some sample sequences in Chapter Eight. You may wish to select poses that target your problem areas, but I also suggest selecting at least one pose from each category to string your own sequence together. Remember that the order isn't set in stone. Always follow your practice with Savasana, the resting pose. Yogic resting is marvelous for the face, and will instantly pay off in the form of a more radiant, unlined complexion. Once you begin this practice, you will find the benefits these poses afford practically addictive. You will begin to crave your daily practice.

Use a yoga mat when you practice so you don't slip and slide. Go barefoot when practicing the standing poses and the balancing poses, so your feet can grip the mat. When you move to the floor for seated poses, inversions, or Savasana, feel free to put socks on. The room temperature should be warm to aid in softening up and lengthening the muscles.

Special Considerations:

If you are pregnant or injured or have high blood pressure, consult with your doctor before embarking on your practice. In general, a healthy pregnancy can be enhanced by practicing yoga, but be mindful about doing deep twists, heart-rate accelerators, and anything on the belly. If you have high blood pressure, avoid lifting your hands at an overhead angle.

Practicing inversions such as handstands, headstands, and shoulderstands depends more on your level of practice before pregnancy. If you were practicing those postures easily before, you can probably continue them through pregnancy. If however, you are a beginner, avoid learning these poses until pregnancy is concluded.

Green/Earth

The earth is associated with vigor, vitality, and strength. The first chakra is often linked with the element of earth, governing physical health and the material plane. A strong connection to the earth, enhanced by practicing these postures, will cultivate health, youthfulness, ease, and lightness in the body, and will translate to the skin as regeneration, increased circulation, and enhanced regeneration of the cells. Skin, hair, nails, and teeth are all associated with the earth element and its corresponding chakra, Muladhara. Practicing these poses will improve their strength and appearance. Being steady and firm on the earth through standing and balancing will keep your face relaxed and your jaw released.

These poses are divided into two categories: Balancing Poses and Standing Poses.

Balancing Poses

Balance is strength, and all your muscles must coordinate to meet the challenge. Draw strength from the earth with the soles of your feet, and then draw your energy into the center line of your body when performing a balance. The key to balance is also a metaphor for life: it's all about focus. Pick a focal point (in Sanskrit, *drishti*) upon which to gaze, preferably a stationary object in your horizon line (more advanced: the tip of the nose, or eyes closed). Keep the focus as unwavering as possible. As in life, you will surprise yourself by what you achieve when you keep it simple and focus. Training your gaze to be specific but not too intense and keeping your focus sharp but released is a great practice for toning the oculus orbus muscles, the ring muscles around the eyes. If you can train yourself in the challenging asanas to keep a smooth, steady gaze, devoid of furrowing and wrinkling (which signifies too much effort and paradoxically will make it easier for you to lose your balance, as you are gripping too much and are therefore rigid), you will train your facial muscles to stay released and calm at all times.

Balancing poses will take stress and gripping away from the facial muscles as well—facial releasing translates to a smoother, less furrowed brow and a looser jaw. These poses fight marionette lines (the lines that form between the mouth and the nose, like those of a puppet).

Standing Poses

Standing poses require concentration but must not be performed with too much effort or the face will clench and tighten. The balancing in standing poses teaches us to maintain our serenity and a relaxed facial demeanor in the face—pun intended—of a challenge. Doing them is a great way to practice grace under pressure, and they will train the facial muscles to stay smooth and unruffled in stressful situations. If you are prone to worrying, doing these poses is an excellent way to counter the stress and worry lines around your forehead, eyes, and mouth. They encourage the facial muscles to relax.

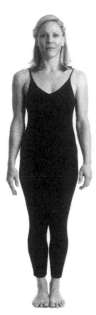

Mountain Pose (Tadasana)

This is the foundation of all the other poses: elements of this pose can be found in all of the asanas. It is like first position in ballet and is a simple, stable, extremely grounding pose that you can practice anywhere, anytime. Placing yourself in Tadasana for five minutes can be a calming yet energizing experience, a standing meditation. Emotionally this pose teaches us to be strong and steady, focused and calm. It gives a lot of earth energy, which enhances the health of the skin and hair and reminds us that being still and doing "nothing" can be a potent form of action.

Stand with the middle lines of your feet parallel, the big toe joints touching. Look at the outer edges of your feet and try to make them parallel, too. Lift the crown of your head up on top of your spine. Close your eyes and feel your collarbones broadening and your shoulder blades spreading like wings on your back. Drop the bottom tips of your shoulder blades down toward your waist. Externally rotate your upper arm bones slightly while internally rotating your forearms, turning your palms in toward your thighs. Lift your rib cage up off your pelvis. Visualize, then drop your pubic bone down toward the inner arches of your feet. Curl the bottom of your tailbone slightly under you and also toward the mid-arches of your feet. Plant your heels down on the floor and feel your pelvis and lower back becoming more open and spacious.

Next, plant the balls of your feet down. Try rolling to the outer edges of your feet, then the inner edges. Rock to the balls of your feet, then the heels. Finally, find your most grounded, even stance by pressing all four corners of your feet on the ground evenly. Breathe deeply, and feel your stance, strong, tall, and easy. Do not lock your knees. Visualize the earth's energy (you can imagine it as a specific color—perhaps green—if you like) running up the front of your body through the soles of your feet, into your calves and thighs, through your pelvis, torso, and heart, up to the crown of your head and then down the back of your body, back into the earth. Visualize this cycle several times. Breathe into the back body, especially filling up the kidneys and then the lungs with air. Savor the strength and ease of being in your body, firmly rooted in the earth.

While standing like this, close your eyes and imagine your face. De-wrinkle it by breathing and letting tension go. Imagine your brow smooth and unlined. Unclench your jaw. Relax your eyes, and imagine them sinking deeply back into their sockets. Smile lightly. Your face will loosen its grip and the jaw will release, preventing forehead wrinkles and pucker lines around your mouth. Smile and breathe contentment. This pose can take five to fifteen minutes.

Warrior 2

Although it is numerically the second warrior pose, Warrior 2 is an easier pose to start your practice with than Warrior 1, so I list it first.

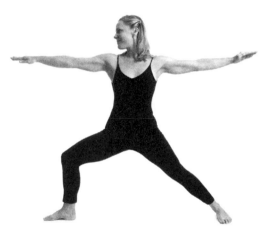

This pose opens up the hips, pelvis, lower back, shoulders, and upper back. It also strengthens the thighs and buttocks. It creates room for the internal organs to breathe and thereby detoxifies the system, creating a more youthful appearance. It lends a sense of strength, stability, freedom, ease, and flexibility. Runners and walkers should always do this stretch after a workout. Practiced with a gentle smile and your teeth separated from one another lightly, this pose will release jaw tension and smooth frown lines.

Start on the right side, with the right foot facing forward and the left foot perpendicular to the right, about four feet behind. Adhere the outer edge of the back foot firmly to the floor; though in the beginning this may feel challenging, over time you will make progress. Bend the front knee so that the front thigh is parallel to the floor, with the right knee in direct alignment over the right ankle—not in front of, or behind it. Open the hips sideways (toward the left side when your right foot is forward) and bring your spine as vertically centered over the hips as possible. Do your best to keep the arms extended over the legs and parallel to the floor, and avoid the tendency to drop your back hand lower than your front. Allow the crown of your head to float on top of the spine, and smile. Breathe into the lungs and feel the back ribs expand as you extend the breath. Take five to eight counts here. Then, switch sides.

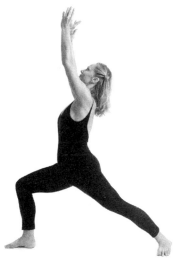

Warrior I

Start with feet about hip-width apart. Step forward in a lunge (right foot forward first). Turn down your left heel to a 33-degree angle. The back heel may not press down completely right away—that's okay. Over time you will see progress. Lift your arms above your head, turning your palms to face each other shoulder-width apart or pressing together in prayer. Lift your sternum toward the ceiling. Drop the bottom tips of your shoulder blades down your back toward your waist. Press your left hip point forward and draw your right hip back. Continue to bend your right knee deeply (make sure the knee doesn't extend out in front of the ankle in the lunge, however—it should be on top, in a 90-degree angle, and not in front). Hold this pose for five to eight long breaths, then repeat on the other side, with the left foot forward.

· · ·

The warrior poses open up the body to receive grounding earth energy, and they free up the heart, kidneys, and lungs, allowing for increased circulation to the face. When your heart receives more circulation, more oxygen goes to the blood cells and, in turn, the skin.

Warrior 3

A challenging balancing pose as well as a standing pose, this pose aligns the heart and the head at the same level. The skin of the face receives more oxygen, so this pose will enhance and improve skin tone. Because this pose is challenging and requires a lot of concentration, it is a great way to

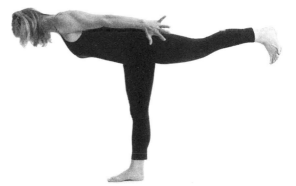

practice grace under pressure. Try smiling in this pose, and etch your muscle memory with a template of facial relaxation even when you'd normally scowl and tighten. This will translate into a smoother, more wrinkle-free countenance no matter what the outer circumstances. This pose is especially good for de-wrinkling the brows and forehead.

From Tadasana (standing pose), separate your feet hip-width apart and make sure they are parallel. Bend your right knee a little, and extend your hands alongside your hips, palms facing the thighs. Tip your torso forward and pick up your left foot. Turn the left toes down and flex the left foot strongly, and extend your left leg back behind you until the leg parallels the floor. Inner rotate the left thigh and square the hips (i.e., face both hip points toward the floor as evenly as possible). Extend your spine forward and look straight down, either to the floor or to the tip of your nose. Pull the lower abdomen (two inches under the navel) in and up to engage your core muscles, which will help your balance. Your head should be in line with the rest of the spine, but will probably want to tip up a bit. Don't let it. Hold this pose for five counts, if you can. You may struggle with your balance and that's okay! Try the other leg. Do each side once, or if you really enjoy this pose try each side twice.

Do not feel as though you have to completely straighten either the standing or the elevated leg; the standing leg can be a little soft in the knee if you are especially tight in your hamstrings. You can do this pose at the wall by facing the wall and lifting a leg parallel to the floor (full footprint on the wall, toes facing up), then turning away from the wall with the leg parallel to the floor and turning the foot on the wall so that the toes point down. Beginners or those experiencing physical challenges may wish to use a chair to aid in balance—lean on the same side arm as the leg that's lifting up the wall on the chair back.

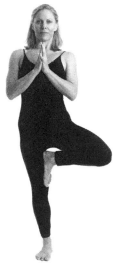

Tree Pose

Tree pose encourages external rotation of the thighs, releasing pent-up emotions that constrict and tighten the face. It also stretches the hip flexors while encouraging balance and strength. Imagine that your standing leg has roots connected from the sole of the foot to the center of the earth, and envision your trunk and limbs growing out of this rooted foundation. Bonus: try Tree with your eyes closed, once you have set up the stance, and try to find your inner balance. Contrary to what

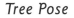

many of us think, it's not our eyesight that gives us our sense of balance. Balance is perceived from deep within our core and also corresponds to the inner ears.

Stand on your right leg and bend the knee of the left leg outward, away from your pelvis. Bring the left foot to the right inner thigh or calf. Place your palms in prayer position at the center of your chest and smile. If you like, you can practice Lion Face simultaneously: scrunch all your facial muscles on an inhale, then exhale and stick out your tongue and roll your eyes. Not only will Lion Face give you a total facial stretch, doing it while in Tree Pose will increase your concentration and balance. Hold for five to eight counts, then switch sides.

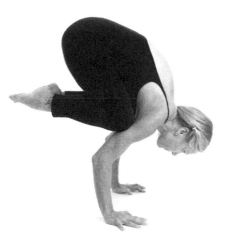

Crow Pose

Crow is a great inversion, meaning the head is lower than the heart, and the face receives freshly oxygenated blood. You will emerge from Crow facially radiant and glowing. If you are prone to bags and hollows under the eyes, this pose is an antidote.

Squat down, and press your hands shoulder-width apart on the floor with a wide hand spread. Draw your shoulders down your back and lift your navel up toward your spine. Lift and press one knee at a time behind your upper arms, rounding your upper back and letting your big toes touch. Try to lift both feet off the floor. Look down and slightly forward. Place a pillow or blanket on the ground beneath your head in case you roll forward. If you do fall, tuck and roll!

Hold this pose as long as you can. For most people this is going to be rather fleeting, but ideally, a count of five is a good place to start. Once you are more proficient with this pose, try holding for ten counts. Try it two times.

Blue/Water

Energy regulating, receptive, cooling, and relaxing, the water poses help to regulate moisture by hydrating what is dry and reducing puffiness where needed. I have divided the blue poses into several categories: Contemplatives, Forward Bends, Hip Openers, and the ultimate resting pose, Savasana.

Contemplative Poses

Contemplative poses are excellent for those suffering from wrinkles around the eyes or the forehead. If you practice daily for three to five minutes, it will smooth these areas.

Any time you experience serenity, your face will automatically reflect this quality. The experience of facial releasing in the Contemplatives will become a part of your muscle memory for other situations where you are under pressure. This will reduce your tendencies to clutch, grip, and etch worry lines onto your face. If you are prone to anxiety or insomnia, you should practice these poses often.

Buddha Face

Practice cultivating a smooth, sweet face while sitting peacefully. Close your eyes or keep your eyes softly open and smile slightly. Buddha face can also be practiced while you are in any other pose. Hold for ten to twenty counts.

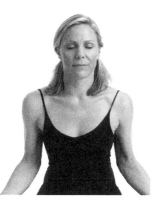

Easy Pose (Sukhasana)

This pose will help you cultivate a smooth, wrinkle-free face as you release stress and the muscular habits of clenching and gripping. Training your facial muscle memory to be free and loose, you will let go of worry and the unattractive wrinkles it causes.

The word *asana* is translated as "seat." The Yoga Sutras of Patanjali, the basic philosophical yoga text, tell us that the asana should be steady and comfortable, and Easy Pose is just that.

While seated, let your knees drop lower than your hips if possible. You may use padding—in the form off a rolled-up blanket or a yoga block—under the sit bones to make it more comfortable.

Sitting in a chair or on a couch is a good alternative to Easy Pose for beginners. You may wish to insert a columnlike pillow, bolster, or rolled-up blanket behind your spine to encourage your posture. Draw your shoulders back, broaden your collarbones, and allow the crown of your head to float on top of the spine. Keep your gaze forward or on the tip of your nose. Rest your dominant hand in your passive one, both hands facing up, and breathe steadily and smoothly. Practice this for two or three minutes, minimum, or choose it as a meditative seat and sit as long as you can—up to twenty or thirty minutes if possible—in meditation.

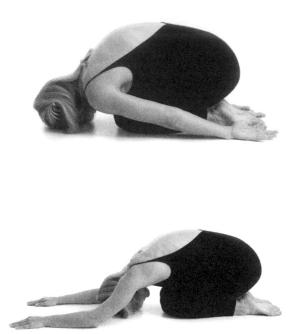

Child's Pose

Child's Pose is the perfect posture for erasing worry lines from the face. Your head is dropped lower than your heart, so the face can receive more circulation. It stretches the back and drains away the excess fire and aggression that can make unattractive scowl and worry lines appear between the eyebrows and on the forehead. Choose either variation.

Drop down on the floor, knees bent, and rest your front ribs on the tops of the thighs. Place a pillow or block under your forehead if it doesn't reach the floor. You can put a pillow or rolled-up blanket between your heels and buttocks if there is a gap between them. Extend your arms forward, palms down, or alongside your torso, palms up. Hold this pose for about ten deep breaths.

Threading the Needle

This pose is a variation of Child's Pose that also stretches the neck, jaw, shoulders, and arms and is therefore a heart-opening pose, bringing increased circulation to the face and detoxifying the lymph nodes. From Child's Pose, thread your left arm under your collarbones, face up toward the right. Turn on the left side of your face, resting on the left side of the head.

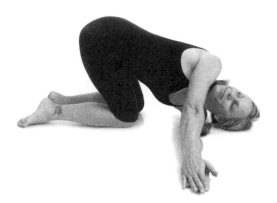

Stack your right palm on top of your left so that your hands meet in prayer, perpendicular to your torso. Come back to Child's Pose, repeat on the other side. Hold for five counts on each side.

Forward Bends

Forward bends are the yogic equivalent of coming home. Inward and self-reflective, they are cooling and restorative. They embody the yogic concept of pratyahara (withdrawal) to draw in the senses. If you are in need of space, try these poses. If you are constantly around others, you will find these poses especially soothing. Forward bends also encourage the face to drop, so that you may receive more oxygen and blood in the head. This translates to a rosier complexion and a less gaunt face. Forward bends also prevent and correct facial hollows that can develop with age.

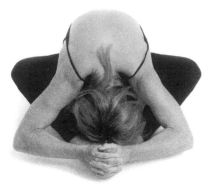

Star Pose (Tarasana)

In this pose, the head drops lower than the heart again and receives the blessing of new circulation. The heart rate slows, the back, hips, and gluteal muscles are stretched, and the face projects a rosy, dewy glow. Sit down, place the soles of your feet together, and bend your knees outward. Your legs should resemble the shape of a baseball diamond. Grab your shins, ankles, or the tops of your feet, bend your elbows out to the sides, and drop your head as low as you can. Rounding your upper back a little here is fine, but release the bottom tips of your shoulder blades toward your waist gently if you can. Hold this pose for five to ten counts.

Seated Forward Bend (Paschimoltanasana)

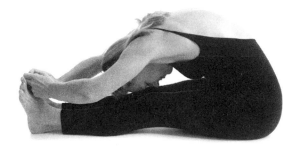

Deep forward bends take years off the face, as they ease strain and tension and drop the head lower than the heart. The ultimate forward bend, Paschimoltanasana (or "East Meets West Pose") lengthens the upper and lower back, hamstrings, and calves. Sit on your mat, legs extended in front of you. Engage your quadriceps (the tops of the thighs) without locking your knees. Pick up the flesh outside the thighs and roll it—along with the thighs—toward the midline to encourage inner rotation of the thighs, which will release the lower back. On an inhale, extend your arms upward, hands shoulder-width apart and facing each other, and as you exhale, reach your fingertips toward your toes. Grab your shins or place your palms down on the floor alongside the knees or shins if you are unable to touch the toes. If you can go deeper in the stretch, try to grab the outer edges of your feet. On your next inhale, arch the upper back a little, and slightly bend your elbows out to the sides to release the shoulders down the back and broaden the collarbones. Avoid rounding the upper back, as this shortens the lower back muscles. Try to go for a flat back instead of a rounded back. Then, release the face toward the legs and take eight slow, deep breaths. To make this pose more calming and restful, roll a blanket into a long cylinder and place it on top of the legs, and then rest your forehead on top of the blanket. Add one or two more blankets if one isn't enough.

If you are tight in the back and/or hamstrings, sit on a rolled-up blanket to lighten the pressure. You may also make your hands into fists and bend your elbows to create a 90-degree angle in the forearms. This will release the antagonist muscles in the lower back. If you are prone to hyperextension, bend your knees a little or place a rolled-up blanket under the backs of your knees. Breathe deeply and mindfully. We tend to breathe less deeply in forward bends, as though we have forgotten to nourish ourselves. This is when breath matters most!

Hip Openers

Hip opening poses help to unlock repressed emotions. Yogic folklore says that the hips are the receptacles for forbidden or taboo emotions such as rage and excessive passion. You may feel both an emotional and a physical load lifted in these poses, but also be prepared to really feel your feelings here. The jaw will want to clamp down, repressing the anger or sadness that wants to release, so it is important to let the jaw relax. You can flutter your lips or open the mouth and say *aaaaah* while in a hip opening posture. This will release tension from the face instantly.

Let yourself breathe into these poses, be present to any emotions that come up, and let stress wash out of you on the exhale. Your mind may panic in a hip opener, telling you too much is coming up. But these poses are powerful precisely because they can bring us to a new level of feeling. When the hip flexors are stretched, the lower back feels better. Leg extension improves. Forward bends are easier. Walking feels delicious. There is an ease, spaciousness, and grace in movement. Your face will look lighter and less tense. Mindfully relax your face as your hips relax to combat jaw clenching, marionette lines, and wrinkles in the brow and forehead.

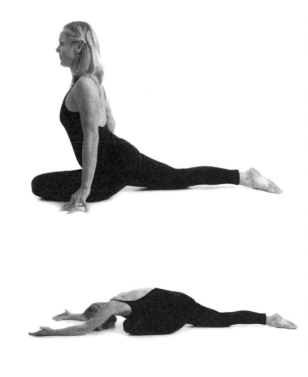

Pigeon Pose
(Eka Pada Rajakapotasana)

A surrendering pose, Pigeon improves circulation in the face and erases worry lines. It also stretches the gluteal muscles and the hip flexors. As a forward bend, this pose opens up the channels for restoration of energy.

On your mat, place your right knee between your hands, which should be spaced shoulder-width apart, as your left leg extends back behind you, with the left knee toward the midline of the mat. Draw your right ankle and shin toward your left wrist, but only as far as you can comfortably. You will feel this in the buttocks and outer upper thigh. Walk your hands backward toward your hips on fingertips until you bracket your hips with your hands. On an inhale, curl your tailbone under you, draw in the navel, and lift the upper chest. Bend the elbows slightly backward toward your waist to draw the shoulder blades down the back and expand the collarbones. As you exhale, walk your hand back out in front of your head and place your palms or fingertips on the floor. Turn the palms up, shoulder-width apart, to create more release in the shoulders. Rest the forehead on the floor or on a block or blanket. Breathe deeply for eight counts. Then repeat this on the other side. Do once on each side.

Open Angle Pose
(Upavista Konasana)

This pose clears the channel of energy from the tail to the crown, allowing the kundalini (energy of enlightenment) to travel unimpeded. Keep the heart open

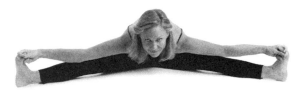

and the shoulders released. This pose releases tension from the hip flexors and releases trapped negative emotions, such as fear, anxiety, and anger, from the face, leaving joy to shine through the facial features. It also strengthens the thighs and stretches the hip flexors and hamstrings.

Sitting on your mat, extend your legs into a wide V shape. Externally rotate your thighs by lightly pulling the flesh out from under them and rolling the thigh bones in toward the midline. Flex your feet and engage your quadriceps, then open the arms wide as though you wished to hug the world. Lead from the sternum and reach for the tips of the big toes or the outer edges of your feet. Don't worry if you don't make contact. If you don't, you can place a block under your forehead, or clamp a block between your hands and slide it forward as flexibility permits. It's a process. Press the backs of your thighs into the floor under you and continue to reach the sternum forward. Smile and breathe deeply for eight slow counts.

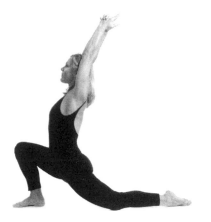

Crescent Moon Pose (Chandrasana)

Lovely and strong, this pose's qualities will translate to your body, mind, and face. The jaw will relax here, especially if you let your teeth part and your tongue release down to the bottom of your mouth and smile. You can even sigh audibly or stick out your tongue to release your jaw. The heart is open, the abdominal and lower back muscles are engaged, and the hip flexors receive stretching. Lift up the back ribs as you go deeper into the back bend. Enjoy the grace!

Support your weight on your right foot and your left knee. Your right foot should fall directly under your right knee. Start by placing your palms down on the right knee and lifting up the spine. Push off the palms to lift the sternum. Tuck the bottom tip of the tailbone slightly under you and pull the lower abdominals in. Arch the upper back. Now step the right foot a little farther forward, perhaps an inch or two, and drop the hips forward. You can interlace your fingers and reach the arms up for a deeper stretch. Hold for about five to eight counts, then switch sides.

The Great Relaxer

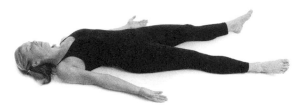

Corpse Pose (Savasana)

Corpse Pose is the traditional ending pose
to asana practice. It is said to emulate the
best aspects of death: letting go, surrender, and cessation of struggle. It is a marvelous
reward to the effort of practice, like dessert after vegetables, but it may also be practiced
anytime, anywhere, on its own merit. Savasana reduces facial puffiness and bloating. Really let go of facial tension here, as it is good relaxation training for your facial muscles.

The face receives maximum benefit from this pose. Savasana is not heavy slumber; rather, it is a light, restful state in which no grogginess takes place. The jaw releases, the mouth softens, the forehead unfurrows.

Lie down with your feet hip-width apart and your hands palms-up alongside your
hips. Let your back body drop into the floor. Close your eyes. If you wish, you may cover
your eyes with a scented pillow—lavender is especially soothing. Let your tongue drop to
the floor of your jaw and let your jaw relax. Let your eyes drop to the back of their sockets. Relax completely.

Make sure you are comfortable in this pose; you can roll a blanket (or several to
create a mild inversion) into a long cylinder and place it under your knees to alleviate
back pain. You will experience a deeper relaxation if you are warm, so use an extra
blanket to swaddle yourself if you are not perfectly warm.

After coming out of Savasana, you might like to give yourself a face massage. See
Chapter Four for suggestions.

After a period of rest, you may come back to sitting and meditate. Your mind will
be extremely receptive. Rest in Savasana for a minimum of five minutes; twenty is ideal.

Silver/Air

Rapid and mercurial, air is associated with communication and self-expression. It is also associated with the mental plane: thoughts give rise to action and are then manifested in the physical realm. The realm of air is ethereal. Intuition and precognition are associated with air. Practicing the poses in this category will help you transform your physical reality quickly and easily. These poses will literally turn you upside down and help you let go of preconceptions and fixed ideas about who you are and how you appear. A well-performed inversion often gives us the sense of being able to transcend physical boundaries. Air is associated with speech and speaking, and corresponds physically to the throat, neck, lips, and cheeks. These poses will help to tone and invigorate these facial regions.

Inversions

Inversions enhance facial radiance, fill facial hollows, and regulate the thyroid and other glandular functions. The thyroid is an important regulator of hormonal function, and when imbalanced it can negatively affect metabolic function, which can cause swelling and bloating around the face and neck, along with unnecessary weight gain and water retention. The pituitary and hypothalamus are stimulated in head balances such as Headstand, which helps to keep youthful energy flowing and bring radiance to the face.

When the head is lower than the heart in inversion practice, the heart rate slows and the brain and face receive more oxygen, which counters the rapid acceleration associated with aging. For example, a night of insomnia ravages the face. When I suffered from insomnia, I noticed that I had large rings and bags under my eyes. Practicing inversions helped me sleep better and has noticeably rejuvenated my facial appearance.

Inversions are mega-anti-agers. They give the face a rosy glow. Inversions plump the skin and fill in sags and bags. However, avoid these poses if you have high blood pressure or if you are pregnant.

Plow Pose (Halasana)

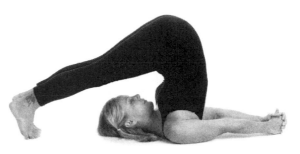

Your face will get a huge shot of energy and life force when the chin locks to the sternum (in Sanksrit, Jalandhara Bandha, or "capping off," lock, so called because it reverses the downward flow of energy and sends life force back up to the upper body, neck, and face) here. It brings oxygen and color to the face, and firms the throat, neck, and chin. Plow Pose is a detoxifier and a wonderful back stretch. It can also be thought of as an upside-down forward bend, and is a great alternative to Seated Forward Bend for those with tight hamstrings, as gravity helps to deepen the forward bend without pulling on the leg muscles.

Lie down on your back, palms facing down alongside your legs, and lift your legs over your head. Walk your arms under your back toward your spine, and interlace your hands. Walk your feet as far away from your head as possible, then roll your shoulders under your back. Enjoy Jalandhara Bandha lock here. You can try pointing your toes and engaging your thigh muscles, or you may flex your feet to feel the stretch more in the hamstrings.

Handstand (Adho Mukha Vrksasana)

Not everyone can, or wishes, to practice handstands, but if you are willing to try, you may find them extremely rejuvenating. They require strength and coordination as well as bravery. By literally turning yourself upside down, you will receive all the beauty and anti-aging benefits of inversion, plus an extra dollop of grace. As an inversion, a handstand lets the face receive freshly oxygenated blood. Handstand connects us to playfulness and the joyfulness of youth—the inner kid comes out to play. You'll see your cares leave your face. If you are prone to bags and hollows, this pose is an antidote.

Start from a Downward-Facing Dog position (see page 72) facing a wall with your hands shoulder-width apart. Make sure you have eight to ten inches between the wall and your hands. Lift up one leg very slowly, keeping your hips as square as possible, then lift the other leg up to meet the first. You may need someone to spot you on this pose, or try it in a class with an experienced teacher before doing it at home by yourself. Rest in Child's Pose after your handstand for five breaths.

To try a handstand off the wall, follow the steps for practicing at the wall, then lift one leg at a time away from the wall. Flex each foot strongly as it leaves the wall, and when both are in the air, draw the inner thighs in toward one another and drop the head between the upper arms, crown facing down, rather than arching the neck and looking up. Tuck the tailbone under, and draw the pubic bone toward the tail to broaden the lower back and engage the abdominal muscles. Draw the front ribs in toward the spine rather than letting them arch, which will compress the lower back and take you out of alignment. Remember, this is called "upside-down tree" in Sanskrit, so you want to use the same

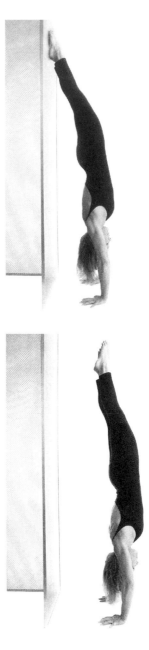

principles of standing upright, only upside down. If you feel unstable, touch your feet back to the wall, then drop one leg at a time back to the floor and rest for five breaths in Child's Pose.

Hold this pose for as long as you can. But save some energy to dismount with precision. Five to ten counts is a good place to start.

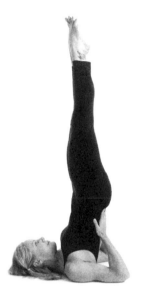

Shoulderstand (Sarvangasana)

Called the queen of the poses by the sages, this pose is a true yogic facelift. It reverses sagging skin and brings a luminous quality to the skin and the eyes. It removes eye rings and hollows. As a direct conduit to lunar energy, it removes excess aggression and slows the heart rate, deaccelerating the aging process. The chin tucks into the sternum (Jalandhara Bandha), sealing vital energy (prana) into the upper chamber of the chest. The Jalandhara Bandha lock redirects downward-flowing energy back up to the heart, lungs, brain, and face, which provides a youthful rejuvenation and gives you a brilliant, luminous face.

This pose is said to help regulate the thyroid gland and the rest of the endocrine system. Be mindful of this pose's power, and avoid practicing it when menstruating or pregnant (you may practice Legs-Up-the-Wall—the following exercise—instead).

Take a blanket and fold it in half, or quarters, making sure it has no ripples or bulges. Place the blanket one third of the way down your mat, the upper portion of the mat above the blanket. Lie down with your head over the edge of the blanket, and roll your shoulders toward each other. Bring your upper arm bones under your back toward the midline as much as you can. Make sure you are not resting weight on the vertebra at the base of your cervical spine, where it attaches the neck to the shoulders (the C7 vertebra). You should feel that vertebra tucking in and up in the direction of the front of the throat. There should be a hollow under your neck at this point, and a bit of a curve. When you have ascertained that these points of alignment are in place, interlace the fingers under your back and draw the palms toward each other to make one fist. Walk the legs over the head, and extend the arms and hands in the opposite direction, away from the tailbone. Then, roll your shoulders under you again, and take the palms to the back, tucking the elbows toward each other in the middle of the mat. Lift up one leg, and then the other. Now, inner rotate the thighbones and press the thighs slightly away from the face. Flex your feet overhead to energize them, then you can arch the feet and flare the toes toward your face like Barbie feet. Press the pelvis slightly toward your face. If possible, walk your palms (fingers pointing toward the tailbone) higher up your back toward the shoulder blades. You should feel light and effortless here, with no pressure on the cervical spine. If you do feel pressure on the cervical spine, back off and practice Vipariti Karani ("Legs-Up-the-Wall," the next posture) instead. If it feels good, take your gaze to the breastbone and count twenty slow, deep breaths, then lower the legs over the head, and take the hands in the opposite direction for Plow (Halasana), then press the palms down toward the bottom of the mat and use your hands for brakes as you roll from the top of the spine to the bottom one vertebra at a time, until you reach the floor. Take this "dismount" from the pose very slowly, and use your abdominal muscles to control the descent.

Legs-Up-the-Wall Pose (Vipariti Karani)

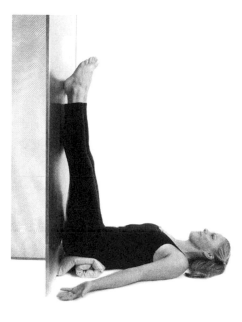

Vipariti Karani is a mild inversion that gives you the same benefits (to a lesser degree) as Shoulderstand without the same physical challenges. I recommend it for beginners and those with physical limitations that preclude practicing Shoulderstand (such as neck injuries or shoulder tightness). It is calming, reverses the downward flow of energy, and brings your prana (life force) back up to the upper chest, neck, throat, and face, endowing you with a rosy glow and slowing the heart rate.

Sit sideways at a wall, with your knees bent and right hip touching the wall. Recline and lift your legs up the wall. Table-top your legs by pressing the feet hip-width apart into the wall and pushing your pelvis toward your face, hands on the floor for support. Slide a rolled-up blanket or a block under your sacrum, drop your lower back on your support, and lift your legs straight up the wall. You may cover your eyes with a scented pillow for enhanced relaxation. As an option, you can spread your legs wider and enjoy the hip opening! Stay here for three to five minutes, minimum. You can go up to ten minutes for super-rejuvenating effects.

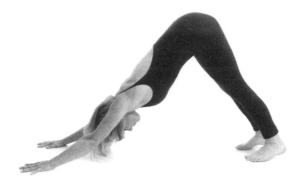

Downward-Facing Dog (Adho Mukha Svanasana)

A great strengthener and lengthener, Downward-Facing Dog stretches the calves, hamstrings, lower and middle back, spine, and shoulders. It builds strength in the arms, shoulders, abdominals, and quadriceps, and provides a nice inversion. Do not be discouraged if this pose feels challenging. Like all the poses, it takes a while to develop openness and flexibility here. Keep breathing and enjoy the feeling of length and release.

From Child's Pose, come on to the hands and knees. Tuck your toes under you, and lift the hips up, as you walk your hands about two feet forward, shoulder-width apart. Walk your legs back, and make sure the feet are hip-width apart and parallel to the best of your ability. Look at the fingers, and make sure the thumb and index are wide apart, and center the middle fingers to face the top of the mat and keep them parallel to one another. Let your neck be released, and draw in the front ribs toward the center of the spine. Then, look at your navel or between your upper thighs as you hold the pose. Think of this pose as an equilateral triangle, with the floor being one side, your hips, pelvis, and legs the second side, and the torso, arms, and head the third side. Don't bog your front body down with your weight. Keep the legs active by engaging the quadriceps (front of the thigh muscles), but avoid locking the knees. Don't worry if your heels don't reach the floor right away. Like all the poses, this pose takes years to really master and the journey is as important as the destination. Try to rotate the upper arm bones outward, and drop the bottom tips of the shoulder blades down your back toward your waistline. Bring the upper arm bones into their sockets. Inhale and engage the muscles, exhale and release. At the bottom of the exhale, draw your sit bones toward each other and gently pull the navel into the spine. Hold this pose for eight breaths if possible. You can pedal your feet out for a few breaths first, stretching through the Achilles tendon and the calves to warm up, before reaching the heels down together.

Modifications: if you are tight in the legs, slightly bend your knees. Do not jam your knee joints or lock them, as this will lead to hyperextension. Engage your quadriceps but leave your knees as loose and open as possible. Do not worry if your heels don't touch the ground. The act of reaching for something is part of the process, and if the pose is not challenging enough, walk your legs back an inch or so farther. You can place a yoga prop block under your crown or forehead to stimulate the crown center, which will aid in sending oxygen to your face and slow down your heart rate.

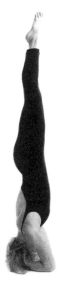

Headstand (Sirsasana)

Headstand is the king of poses. The counterpart to Shoulderstand, Headstand is radiantly energetic and solar in nature. This is actually a fire pose, but since it is an inversion, I have included it here. Headstand stimulates the pituitary gland, which governs blood pressure, and regulates water in the body, metabolism, some sex organ functions, and thyroid function. Kneel down, interlace your fingers behind the back of your head and bend over, placing your forearms shoulder-width apart on the floor. You may do this at a wall in the beginning, allowing your knuckles to line up into the wall. "Down dog" your legs and walk your feet in toward your head. Push firmly down into your forearms, and draw your shoulders away from your ears. Engage your lower abdominals, and use your core strength to lift your legs up, one at a time, into the pose. Hold five to ten breaths.

To ready yourself for Headstand, you can simply practice the preparation, bracketing the back of the head with the interlaced fingers, and coming on to the crown of the head as you simulate Downward-Facing Dog in the back and legs. Place a lot of weight and pressure on the inner wrists and forearms so you don't place too much weight on your head and neck. Draw the bottom tips of the shoulders toward each other on your back. Warning: incorrect alignment can lead to compression of the cervical spine—if you are in doubt, take class with an experienced yoga teacher who is used to teaching the basics and make sure you are doing this correctly!

The following mega-poses for the face possess aspects of all the elements. They can be practiced independently of or in conjunction with the others. I have included a color code to indicate their general element and nature.

The Face Lifters

These poses tone the muscles under the skin of the face and throat through specific muscular isolation in the facial area.

Fish Pose (Blue)

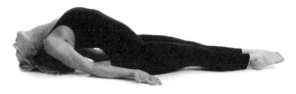

Fish Pose is named after a noble prince who was transformed into a fish so he could learn the various poses. Once he learned them, he resumed his human form and taught his fellow humans the poses. Fish is a beautiful example of total surrender and vulnerability. Opening the heart, throat, face, shoulders, back, and abdomen, Fish Pose helps us to breathe through the side seams, where a fish has gills. This pose is a total release, but it takes strong back muscles. Sit on your mat with your legs extended. Bending at the elbows, arms alongside the hips, lean back and rest weight on the forearms as you arch your back and gently drop the top of your head back toward the floor. If your head doesn't make it all the way down, place a folded blanket or small pillow under the crown to bridge the gap. You can make the shoulders release here by placing one hand at a time palm-up under your respective buttocks, then "walking in" the elbows toward one another under your back. Then, lift your sternum up as you gently drop back the crown of the head toward the floor. Once you have found your alignment, you can slide one palm at a time up and alongside the hips, resting weight on the elbow points. Hold this for five to ten deep breaths. You can roll up a blanket and place it under your shoulder blades perpendicular to your body to provide extra support, alleviating muscular effort. Fish will smooth out the forehead and unclench the jaw. Slide your lower teeth over your upper teeth while relaxing your tongue, to firm the throat, neck, and chin.

Lion Face (Red)

Lion Face is an all-purpose face workout that stretches, tones, and firms all your facial muscles and releases stress. You may find yourself laughing while you do it. That's great!

Scrunch your facial muscles and buttocks and make your hands into fists on an inhale. On the exhale, stick out your tongue, roll your eyes up, and open your hands. Repeat three to four times.

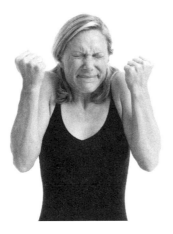 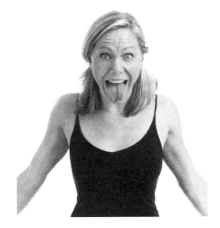

Cat/Cow (Red)

These two poses are usually taught together as a movement sequence. Cat/Cow is a great toner for the facial muscles and throat, and firms the jaw, cheeks, and neck. It stretches the ring muscles around the eye (orbicularis oculi), thereby tightening and firming the skin around the eyes. It lubricates the joints of the spine and will give you more energy and free you of tension.

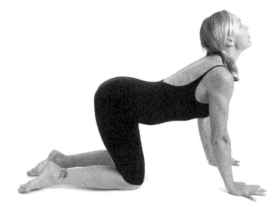

Go on your hands and knees, making sure your wrists are under your shoulders and that your upper arm bones are externally rotating a little to soften the shoulders. Place your knees under your hips. On an inhale, arch your back and look up to the ceiling, stretching your jaw, eyes, throat, and face as you stretch your spine. Then, on an exhale, round your back, still keeping your arms like pillars (the spine, not the arms, should be doing the work here). Repeat three or four times.

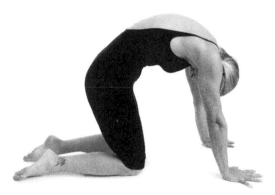

Red/Fire

The element of fire generates heat and reduces lethargy. Fire poses burn off stale energy and toxins, leaving the skin radiant and rosy. Your metabolism will improve through the practice of fire poses. Fire poses are divided into two categories: Back Bends and Detoxifiers, which include Twists and Side Stretches.

Back Bends—Antidepressants

Depression ages the face terribly. It's a vicious cycle: the repeated emotions of sadness trap emotional expressions and etch themselves on the face. We see the sad lines and scowl marks in furrowed brows and marionette lines (the puppetlike lines on the crease between the nose and mouth) around the mouth, and we get more depressed. Then it gets worse, ad infinitum. If we weren't depressed before, one look at a depressed face will make us that way.

Back bends are invigorating, stimulating, and cheerful. They get the heart pumping and include inversion benefits. They release tight hip flexors involuntarily clenched in fear or worry. They, too, work as a facelift.

Back bends benefit the face by bringing a luminescence and rosiness to the skin. Back bends both require and build great strength. They alleviate lower back pain, which releases the face from pinching and wincing. For this reason they are de-wrinklers.

Back bends strengthen the abdominal core, and therefore improve posture, contributing to a slimmer silhouette, which instantly translates to a more youthful appearance (think of the aging effects of stooped, rounded shoulders and hunched backs). Back bends tone the jaw, throat, and neck when the chin is slightly lifted toward the sternum (like a chin-up).

Locust Pose (Salabhasana)

This pose tones the throat and jaw and chin areas. It is a great anti-ager for the whole body because it calls upon the abdominal core muscles and strengthens the muscles and ligaments of the lower and deep back. Locust may feel difficult for you if you aren't accustomed to working this area, but it is a great antidote to lower back pain, and it will tone the tummy. This pose improves posture, and will therefore make you look taller and leaner (instant youth).

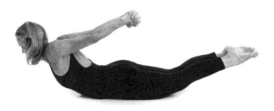

Lie on your belly with your forehead facing down. Place your hands palms-down next to your hips, and bring your big toes to touch as you point your toes and press the tops of your feet down on the floor. Then lift everything up off the floor except your palms—the chest, legs, and head. Gaze down the tip of your nose so you don't strain your neck. Lift your breastbone up toward your chin. Keep your face relaxed and your eyes softly focused on the tip of your nose.

Repeat the exercise, but this time interlace your hands behind your back in a clasp. Or, if that's not comfortable, extend your arms forward, palms facing each other shoulder-width apart and legs about a foot apart, like a flying superhero. Hold each variation for five counts.

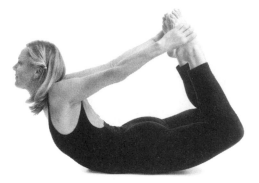

Bow Pose (Dhanurasana)

A magnificent pose for strengthening and toning the back, thighs, and buttocks, this pose also provides an excellent back bend and looks very beautiful. It is definitely an antidepressant, and will carry a sense of beauty and balance into your life. Lift your chest toward your chin to firm the throat, neck, and chin.

Lie on your belly and bend your knees. Grab your ankles, or the tops of the feet. Kick the feet into the hands and lift the legs, head, and chest. Draw the big toes and knees toward each other, unless this hurts your knees. Breathe in and out for five counts. Repeat once again. Smile calmly.

Bridge Pose (Setu Bandha Sarvangasana)

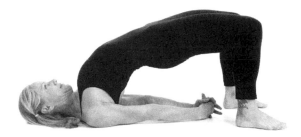

This pose strengthens the lower back and elevates the heart above the head, providing the anti-aging benefits of a mild inversion. It also tones the neck, throat, and chin and is a double-chin preventative or antidote. It will tone the gluteal muscles to give a more shapely appearance to the buttocks. This pose also subverts downward-flowing energy back up to the chest.

Lie down on your back and bend the knees, pressing your feet down on the floor hip-width apart and parallel. Place your palms down alongside the hips. Inhale and lift the pelvis, thighs, and lower back up toward the ceiling. Keep your hips lifted, and walk the arms under the back toward the center of the mat. Interlace your fingers, and press the palms toward each other, shrugging your shoulders toward each other and pressing the chest toward the chin and the chin toward the chest. Press into the inner edges of your feet and your big toes, but keep the knees hip-width apart and parallel. Breathe deeply for five long counts. Take your hands out from under you, and slowly descend from the top of the spine to the bottom, one vertebra at a time, until you are lying down again, feet still on the floor and knees bent. Repeat once or twice. To go deeper, try grabbing your ankles instead of interlacing the fingers under the back, but keep your feet on the floor.

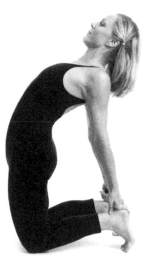

Camel Pose (Ustrasana)

This pose tones the neck, chin, and throat areas. Because this pose lifts the heart higher as the head drops back, the upsurge of heart energy and circulation causes the face to release its customary grips of tension, resulting in a smoother, more relaxed countenance. If you need extra support, you can do this pose with your knees and pelvis at a wall for extra support.

Kneel, legs hip-width apart, and tuck your toes under you. Lift your sternum up and reach back for one heel at a time. Do not drop your head completely back here, as it can hurt the neck. Lift from the center of your chest and gaze up at the ceiling or at your heart. Again, heart lifting causes a slowing down of the heart rate and allows for recirculation, helping energy to flow and giving a youthful glow. When you get more proficient, you may do this pose with your feet flat and toes pointed, away from you. This requires more lower back strength, so approach it with caution.

Detoxifiers

Toxins from stress or diet will accumulate on the surface of the skin. After all, skin is the main excretory organ of the body. It will slough off wastes and impurities through the sweat glands and pores when it can, but it will accumulate what it can't shed on the skin's surface for everyone to see. Age spots, dark circles, rough or scaly patches, dull eyes, and rings under the eyes are all examples of dietary imbalances and toxins appearing on the surface of the skin. The poses that help wring out toxins and stimulate circulation through the internal organs and circulatory system include twists and side stretches.

Twists

Twists are cleansing. They wring out the internal organs like sponges. They improve mental activity, for an aligned and strong spinal column is better equipped to receive and transmit nerve signals to the brain. Twists help create a new sense of perspective: craning your gaze beyond the horizon of your normal view, you perceive new vistas. Twists are stimulating and cleansing. At the foundation, a twist must be rooted and stable in order to be a true twist. Let your eyes twist along with your spine—expanding your focus and stretching your eyes will clear them of toxins and help stretch the ring muscles around the eyes, toning and de-wrinkling them.

Come on, baby let's twist and shout!

Seated Spinal Twist (Ardha Matsyendrasana)

This is a good neck, shoulder, and eye stretch, and very rejuvenating for the face. This pose will help build strength. It also invigorates your thinking power by aligning the spinal column, thereby assisting the nerve signals that conduct to and away from the brain.

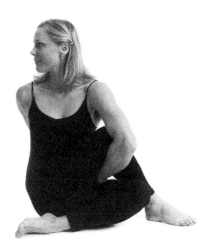

Sit down on your mat. Extend your left leg. Pick up your right leg, and place the right foot, sole down, outside the left knee on the floor. Now bend your left leg, bringing your left foot around to touch your right buttock. Walk your right arm behind your back, and place the right hand palm-down or on the fingertips about six inches or so away from your tailbone, so that your right arm serves as a prop for the spine. On an inhale, extend your left arm up toward the ceiling, and on an exhale, wrap it around your right knee, hugging it in toward your chest. Stay here, and as you inhale lengthen the spine, and as you exhale, twist the gaze, right shoulder, and upper right side of the ribcage to the right. Breathe deeply for five more slow counts. Unwrap the right knee and bring your torso, head, and neck back to center, then counter-twist your spine, head, and neck to the left. Repeat this sequence on the left side.

To modify this pose, extend your lower leg out in a straight line rather than bending the knee and sending the lower leg behind your buttock. If you want to add on a throat, jaw, and chin tightening element to this pose, add the Baby Bird (page 27) while performing this twist.

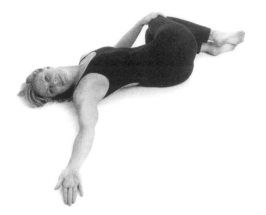

Supine Twist

This pose relieves lower back pain, releases the shoulders, and opens the heart.

Lie down on your back and hug your knees to your chest. Roll your lower back in circles, massaging the lower lumbar area, keeping your shoulder blades on the floor if you can. Then bring your knees back toward the center, then fold them to the left side. Place your left hand on the knees and press down to facilitate the stretch. Extend your right arm and look over your right shoulder. Breathe deeply. Try to reach your right earlobe to the floor. This will release neck and shoulder tension and ease wrinkling in the forehead and between the eyebrows. Come to center, then reverse the twist by moving the bent knees to the right side and looking over your left shoulder. Hold five to eight counts on each side.

Cow Face Pose (Gomukhasana)

This upper arm and shoulder stretch frees up the heart chakra and detoxifies the lymph nodes. For this reason, it is recommended as a breast-cancer preventative. And when you flush your lymphatic system—a major drainage system of the body—toxins will exit rather than show up on your face as dark circles, spots, and bags.

From standing, roll your shoulders a few times first to warm up the area. On an inhale, lift up your right arm, then

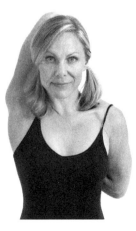

bend at the elbow and drop the hand between your shoulder blades. Take your left arm underneath your shoulder blades from below, and try to walk the fingertips toward each other. Hold for about five deep slow breaths. Take a strap between your hands or the fabric of your shirt to help bridge the gap if you can't bind your hands together. Press your head into your upper arm, and breathe deeply. Repeat on the other side.

Side Stretches

Side stretches help elongate the side seams of the body and also help to strengthen the core abdominals. Side stretches purge the eliminating organs such as the kidneys, liver, intestines, and bladder, thereby purging the face of toxins. This reduces facial bloating and discoloration caused from toxins. If you tend to get "chipmunk cheeks," practice side stretches.

You may feel like you have more room for your internal organs after a good side stretch. Side stretches will also help slenderize the waist. The great yoga master B. K. S. Iyengar calls them "fat burners." By improving the strength of the core, side stretches help alleviate lower back pain. But be careful not to twist the lower back in these poses; rather, twist from above the navel and rotate the ribs in the same direction.

Standing Side Stretch

Stand with your feet together. Steeple your fingers (interlace all but your index fingers, which are pointed skyward) and squeeze the sides of your head with your arms. Lift your ribs and correct the arch in your lower back by tilting your lower back slightly forward, and tucking your tailbone under you. Press your feet down and squeeze your inner thighs together. Then stretch to your right, going as far to the right side from above your navel as you can. Take five deep breaths. Come back up to arms overhead, then stretch to the left.

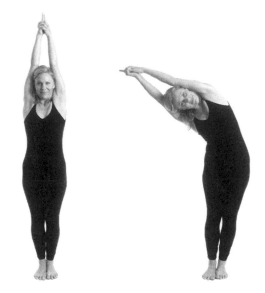

Take five deep breaths. Come back to center and release the arms.

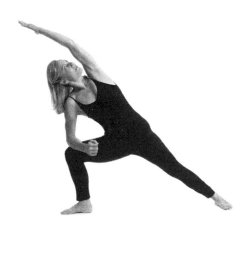

Extended Side Angle Pose
(Utthita Parsvakonasana, modified)

This pose will firm your neck, throat, and jaw and stretch your eyes, de-wrinkling the delicate eye area.

Assume the stance of Warrior 2 (page 51), with your right foot forward. Make your right hand into a fist and prop your elbow on your right thigh like a farmer leaning on a gate. Lift your left arm up toward the ceiling, then angle it over your head. Tuck your chin in toward your breastbone, but direct your eyes to your upper palm. Repeat on the other side. Hold for five to eight breaths.

Gate Pose (Parighasana)

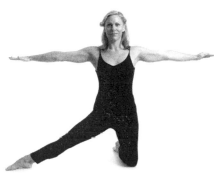

Stretching the side seams of the body helps the organs of elimination (kidneys, bladder, and liver) to receive more circulation, which aids the skin in detoxifying and will impart a clearer, more youthful skin tone. This pose also feels great, as it lengthens and stretches the waist and lower back.

Placing your knees hip-width apart, kneel. If you have sensitive knees, place a folded blanket or towel under them for extra padding. Now extend your right leg out to the right, and maintain a lift in the torso and keep your hips squarely forward. Extend your arms like the wings of an airplane, then tip your right hand down the right shin as you lift your left arm toward the ceiling (left palm facing your ear) and then bend to the right. Lightly brace your right arm on the right shin, keeping your hip points facing forward as best as you can. Hold for six deep breaths. On an inhale, come back up, and then switch sides.

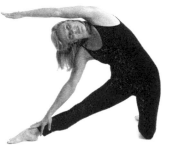

chapter four

Loving Touch

A soft caress can soothe. A brusque tap can annoy. A slap on the back can inspire or alienate, depending on its intensity. Like speech, touch is incredibly varied in what it can communicate, ranging from the subtle to the glaringly obvious.

But have you ever thought about the way you touch yourself? There are countless moments during the day when you make contact with your skin, scrubbing your back in the shower or massaging skin cream into your face. The way you rub your eyes after reading, or maybe when you twist your hair or unconsciously stroke your arms when talking to your boss.

Part of understanding touch is noticing it. And noticing your touch will give you a window into how you relate to yourself. In developing the Yoga Face classes, I started noticing how I treated myself with my touch: I often would apply creams to my face and body hurriedly. I would absentmindedly smear something on my skin while listening to my voice mails. But as I began to be more mindful, I found that I would be more loving to my skin. When I started to pay more attention to my skin by treating it with a loving touch, it got rosier, softer, and smoother.

The facial skin is delicate, and must be treated accordingly. That being said, the popular notion that one mustn't touch one's face for fear of creating wrinkles is wrong. Skin responds well to mindful touch, as this type of touch enhances circulation and frees up energy blocks. Actually, almost everyone craves touch. Massage therapists bank on it. For many, getting a manicure is really an excuse to get some nurturing touch. Touching our own facial skin with the techniques in this chapter is a great way to give ourselves the myriad benefits of massage.

Massage brings many benefits to the skin, including increased circulation, suppleness, and oxygen flow to the tissues. It assists in detoxification, and can break up lactic acid that gathers in the muscles after vigorous exercise. Don't be afraid to touch your skin. You will find that various exercises in this book require different types of touch, from light, feathery, and upward sweeping (to stimulate circulation), to spiraling, pinpoint massage with more pressure. You can be delicate with your fingertips or really bore into a point of tension with your knuckle—it will depend upon the context and your own personal parameters. Always touch your skin with clean hands, and make sure your facial skin is clean and moisturized with whatever oils or creams you like to use (see Chapter Ten for recipes and skin-care products). Start to cultivate a mindful, reverential attitude toward yourself whenever your hands touch any part of your skin.

Acupressure and Massage for the Face, Neck, and Scalp

The ancient art of acupressure spans cultures, but is originally attributed to the Chinese. Chinese medicine puts great stock in acupressure (and its twin, acupuncture), and has evolved a highly sophisticated method of diagnosis and treatment based on pressure points. The overall theory is that energy travels along meridians (like highways in the body), which coalesce in power points all over the body. Nerve endings also travel from point to point, and the organs have energy pathways that end up on the extremities (feet, hands, and face). Many people have become familiar with the acupressure points of the feet (you may have seen the charts hanging in the windows of Chinese massage places) and, to a lesser degree, the hands, but facial acupressure points are still a bit mysterious to Westerners. In this chapter, you will learn how to apply simple acupressure to points on your face, neck, and shoulders to stimulate rejuvenation and release trapped energy.

Warm-up

Start by rolling your head from side to side in half circles. Next roll your shoulders up, back, and down, then reverse directions. Repeat two or three times. Side-stretch your neck on its axis by doing the Sandbag (see page 31). Flutter the lips.

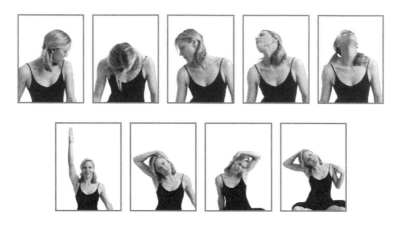

Head, Neck, and Scalp

This sequence can be done in Child's Pose. Gently pick up your head with your fingertips. Using your thumbs, massage the base of your skull, or occipital ridges. Run your thumbs up the outer edges of your neck vertebrae, from the base of the cervical spine to the base of the skull. This ridge, called

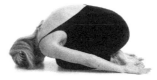

the Pool of Wind in Chinese medicine, is thought to collect energy. Massaging here works to dispel pain and headaches. This point also corresponds to eyesight, and many believe that massaging it will improve vision. Massage for one to two minutes.

Cradle the sides of the skull with your other fingers. Massage the entire scalp as though shampooing your head. Use your fingertips to apply a spiraling, circular touch to the temples, the top of the scalp, and especially the crown.

Crown

In Chinese medicine, this point is called the Junction of One Hundred Channels, through which the body's energy flows. In yoga, your crown center is the highest energetic evolutionary point of all the seven major chakras, the point at which you receive divine inspiration.

Use your middle fingers to rub this point located at the top of the head. This will counter dizziness, headaches, and high blood pressure. It will also stimulate the nervous system. You may also "rake" your fingertips over your skull in ridges to stimulate the scalp, counter tension and headaches, and release accumulated energy. Massage for one to three minutes.

Face

A beautiful way to give yourself a glowing, rosy, supple complexion is to treat yourself to a face massage. You can use either moisturizing cream or a very pure regular oil, not an essential oil (oil containing small amounts of herbs or a floral extract) for massaging. Contrary to what you may have been told, pure oils, when judiciously administered, will not make your skin greasy. They will absorb easily in the skin and leave no residue. Quality is the key here. Because your skin is an organ, and the pores absorb and then transmit what they absorb into the bloodstream, a pure, cold-pressed organic oil such as almond or sesame is preferable to most of the cheaper commercial products that are full of unpronounceable and indecipherable ingredients.

After cleansing your face, lie down, rub a small amount of oil in your hands, and simply start touching the center of your forehead with your fingertips and work outward. Move onto your cheeks, chin, and nose, feeling your facial contours and gently massaging the oil into your skin. Finish the massage by lightly tapping the skin all over your face to allow the pores to drink in the treatment. Massage for two to five minutes.

Jaw Release

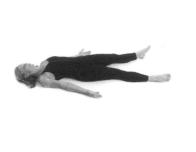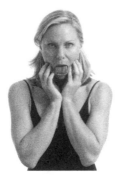

You may do this massage in front of a mirror, but it is more effective if you lie down on the floor in Savasana. Start with your index knuckles below your earlobes and run them in circles from your upper to lower jaw until you reach your chin. Let your lower jaw hang open and drop your tongue to the lower jaw in Slack Jaw. As you go down your jaw with your knuckles spiraling, pay attention to any tight spots and let yourself relax into the massage. Exhale out whatever tension you feel here, or even sigh out a sound of release such as *aaaah*. There is a major pressure point at the hinge between the upper and lower jaw, which is extremely sensitive to some so massage it with caution. If you are prone to clenching or grinding your teeth, you may get great relief from massaging this point. It is common for those who do not openly express anger or desire to clamp up and repress their feelings, and often this manifests as jaw tension.

Pause when you find a sore spot and sigh out a release as you massage it. This helps you let out the emotions that have been causing the tension. I have seen some students cry, yawn, or even laugh as they do this massage. Go with the emotions that come up. As you release your jaw, your eyes will tear and you may begin yawning. This is excellent, as it means you are truly releasing tension and your body is picking up on the release and running with the ball. Yawns help the body take in more oxygen (that's why we yawn when we're tired). They also stretch tense facial muscles. Tearing eyes provide relief from sensory overload, and the tears wash out accumulated environmental toxins. This massage can be from five to ten minutes.

Skull Tap

Make your hands into fists and lightly pummel your skull, like you are tapping a melon. Start from the top of your head and radiate out. This is good for relieving pressure and the energy-sapping effects of technology. Try this massage to refresh yourself after sitting in front of a computer screen. It will bring circulation into your head and scalp and improve your skin color. This should take two minutes or so.

You may also tap your lower back alongside the vertebrae and sacrum, and then continue up the middle back. Try tapping your buttocks, hips, and thighs.

Variation: in a seated posture with your legs extended, tap down the outer legs with your fists, and then tap up the inner legs. Repeat this four times.

Other Face Massage Techniques for Rejuvenation

- **To *unwrinkle the forehead and brow***: Use your knuckles to rub your temples and forehead. Start from the center of your forehead and radiate out to the temples. This massage relieves stress and headaches. Massage for two minutes.
- **To *smooth facial lines and prevent wrinkles*:** A great acupressure point, also helpful for relieving sinus conditions, lies between your nose and your eyes. Press your index fingers or thumbs under the inner arch of your eyebrows, which, again, is helpful for sinus release. Tap the ridge above your eyebrows.
- **To *fight discoloration and bags under the eyes*:** Rub on the point outside of your outer nostrils. Gently rubbing here releases toxins from the body that can show up as blotches and bags under the eyes.
- **To *detoxify and oxygenate the skin*:** Find the apple of your cheeks and press your index finger there.
- **To *free up facial tension*:** Try the Brushing It Off exercise. Place your fingertips in the center of your forehead and sweep outward in horizontal lines. Repeat three times. Now lightly press your palms onto your eye sockets and lightly sweep your fingertips down your cheeks. Repeat three times.
- **To *heighten skin color*:** Pull your middle earlobes out to the sides with your thumb and index finger four times. Grab your lower earlobes and pull down lightly four times. Then grab your upper earlobes and pull up four times. This is an ancient Indian facial yoga technique that brings circulation to the face.

Acupressure and Massage for the Body

The same principles for touching the face apply to the rest of body. Be gentle, loving, and accepting. Do not be overly aggressive. Take the opportunity to celebrate yourself and how good it feels to bask in self-compassion and care. (As with facial massage and acupressure, refer to the sections on cleansing and oils in Chapter Ten to use with the exercises here.)

Hands

Start with the back of your left hand, rubbing the top of the hand with oil and then extending to the fingers. Starting with your pinky and then continuing in toward your thumb, rub at the base of your knuckles a circular motion, then work up the fingers to the middle knuckle and then the fingertips. Pull each finger lightly to release stored-up energy. Then turn the palm up, and work from the outer to the inner palm. There is a major point between the thumb and index finger that corresponds to the intestines. It is also excellent for headache relief. After you have completed the left hand, repeat on the right. Watch for any differences in how you feel in each hand. The left is considered feminine and the right masculine, but being right- or left-handed will also influence how your hands feel. When you have finished both hands, rub them together briskly to generate heat, and place your palms over your eyes, allowing them to drop back in their sockets and absorb the warmth from your hands.

Feet

Reward your feet at night as a special treat after the long day of support they offer. After cleaning your feet (you may soak your feet in the bath or in a basin for ten to twenty minutes—¼ cup Epsom salts mixed with 1 tablespoon baking powder and 2–3 drops lemon or mint oil is especially refreshing for a basin soak), dry them gently, and apply a warmed oil (I like coconut or sesame for hydration and aroma). Rub the tops of your feet first, paying special attention to your toes, and apply spiraling fingertip pressure on the joints connecting the toes to the foot. Then turn your foot over and systematically rub from the top of your foot to the bottom. The pressure points in your feet coordinate with the body from top to bottom, so the points representing your head are at the toes, the middle organs are in the middle of the foot, and so forth. You can also rub your heel area from top to bottom, but be mindful of the reproductive points that are associated with the heel and Achilles tendon; avoid these if you are a woman during your menstrual cycle or pregnancy. After you have massaged your feet, try rolling your feet over a rubber ball (medium-size Kong ball from your local pet store is a good choice) as a method of applying pressure point massage. Stand at a wall, lean back, and place one foot at a time onto the ball. Gently roll back and forth over it, pausing if you find a particularly sensitive spot, and see if you can deepen your breathing and release into the pressure. Once you have finished your foot treatment, drink a nice glass of tea, purified water, or young coconut milk, and put on socks to sleep in so your feet can drink in the oil and your sheets will stay clean. When you wake up, remove the socks and enjoy your baby-soft feet.

Legs

Apply oil to the front and back of your legs. Start with the top of your left leg, with one hand on each side, and make the strokes point toward the center of the leg. Go down the front of the leg and up the back. Repeat on the right leg.

Try standing, feet narrow hip-width apart—five or six inches—and slightly bend your knees so you aren't locking them. Clasp opposite elbows and lightly sway your trunk from side to side. Then let your hands dangle, and bob your knees up and down a few times to shake your legs and loosen your lower back. Then work your fingers from the tops to the bottoms of your legs in a spiraling massage. Start with the front of the legs, moving down, spiraling the fingertips from outward toward the midline (or centerpoint), then go from the upper back thighs to the ankle, again spiraling your fingers from outward toward the midline. You can also "pummel" your legs with your fists. Go from the outer edges of the legs downward, and the inner edges of the legs upward. This massage will take about five to ten minutes.

Swaying Tree

Stand upright, feet parallel and slightly wider than hip-width apart, knees unlocked. Make fists and sway your trunk from side to side, lightly pummeling your buttocks and upper arms. Leading from the swinging of the arms, twist back and forth, keeping your knees bent, and gaining momentum. This is a stimulating and rhythmic exercise, meant to generate energy. It's great for when you're feeling heavy or lethargic.

Knees

The knees are the unsung heroes of the body: they provide amazing structural support and bear a lot of impact, usually with very little complaint. Be good to them, and try this massage: lie down on your back and bend your knees. Hug your right knee to your chest and extend your left leg. Roll the knee in counterclockwise circles. Then, with your thumbs on the kneecap, place your fingertips behind the knee socket and gently run your fingers as if you were playing scales on the piano. Use as much or as little pressure as feels comfortable. You can extend this massage to the back of the calf, the Achilles tendon, and then the foot if you like. Then rub the top of the knees, above the kneecap and below, making a very gentle circular motion with the palm on the kneecap itself. Repeat on the other side. This massage will take about five to ten minutes.

Inner Thighs and Stomach: Goddess Massage

Pamper your inner thighs and stomach with a delightful Goddess Massage. Lie down on your yoga mat or a soft blanket or towel. Place the soles of your feet together and your knees apart. If this places any strain on your knees, you can prop rolled-up blankets, towels, or yoga blocks under your knees—one under each knee. This will take pressure off the knees and lower back.

Start by lightly rubbing oil between your two palms—massage oil scented with sandalwood, with its soothing and relaxing properties would be a nice choice here—and then increase the pressure to heat the oil between your hands. This will release the scent and healing properties of the oil. Place your hands on your hip bones, and gently press down. This will help to release the lower back. Then, feeling your breath rising and falling easily and naturally, begin to very gently rub your inner thighs from their highest point to behind the knees. Use light, feathery strokes. Extend your massage to the tops of your thighs. Rub your knees in a circular motion as well. Massage for five minutes.

Now remove the padding, extend your legs, and go into Savasana. Gently replace the padding under your knees. Place your left hand on your heart and rub your belly in circular motions with your right palm and fingertips. Then close your eyes and rest your hands on your belly and heart.

This is a great way to get in touch with your feminine, receptive energy. Finish with Legs-Up-the-Wall Pose (see page 71) to maximize the calm, relaxing, Goddess Energy. This mild inversion will give the heart and head a circulatory boost.

Lower Back

Because it is hard to access your lower back, massaging the lower back takes using gravity, resistance, and the floor. Add a couple of props into the mix and you're on your way to lower back heaven! (Note: if you have any spinal disk issues, proceed with caution, and make sure you keep your sacral area neutral when taking twists. Twists generally should be performed with the joints above the navel from the middle to upper spine, where they are smaller and are capable of greater mobility. The lower back itself is not built to twist.)

Go into Child's Pose. Rest here and take a deep breath. Then use your hands to gently knead alongside the bones of your lower back. Avoid massaging into any bone directly. Start at the base and see how far up alongside the spine you can go. After a few minutes, switch your touch to light tap-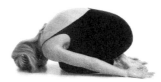ping with easy, loose fists. Try letting out sound on the exhale, saying *aaaaah*.

Then roll over onto your back and hug your knees into your chest. This is a great way to massage the lower back: you have gravity on your side. Place your knees together and your feet about mat-width apart, then cross your arms over your chest, opposite hands on opposite shoulders, and let your spine totally drop into the floor. This is a supportive position—the body exerts no effort to hold itself up here. Try directing the breath into your lower back. Then begin to slowly knock your knees off each another like windshield wiper blades. Then knock them over to the left, extend your arms out, and gaze over your right shoulder. Do this for two to three minutes.

Place your left hand on your outer right thigh, and find the groove below your hip socket with your thumb (it feels like an indentation). Then drag the thumb from the top of your outer thigh to the bottom, giving the ligament that runs outside the thigh (and helps to stabilize the knee) a nice release. Repeat the same sequence on the right side.

Finish with a Happy Baby Pose, in which you grasp your outer feet as you bend your knees to 90-degree angles. Rock back and forth and side to side on your lower back. (Note: if you have difficulty grabbing your outer feet on your own, use a towel or strap to assist you.) This should be a great release for the hip sockets and hamstrings, and rocking from side to side will massage your lower back. Do this for three minutes.

Lastly, "ball up" by hugging your knees to your chest and rock back and forth, exhaling back and inhaling forward, gaining momentum and massaging your entire spine. Rock up to sit, stretch out your legs, lengthen your spine, and take a forward bend (like Seated Forward Bend, page 60). Again, lightly pummel your fists along your spine, this time from top to bottom. Do this for two to three minutes.

Heart Opener

You may wish to play soft music as you do this massage. The sequence will take about ten to fifteen minutes in entirety.

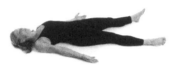

Go into Savasana, arrange any padding (like a rolled-up blanket or blocks) under your knees if you need to relieve pressure in your knees and hips. Lightly oil your hands with massage oil. Place your hands on your heart center, left hand under right. With your eyes closed, listen to your breath. Then softly open your mouth, let your jaw drop down, release your tongue to the floor of the jaw, and make an *aaaaah* sound. Feel the resonation of the sound, letting your body and face relax. Feel the floor supporting the release of your skull, spine, lower back, pelvis, legs, and feet, and continue making the *aaaaah* sound. This is a heart-opening sound, and will help you feel very grounded and energized. It will de-wrinkle and unline the face marvelously. You can experiment with the pitch and duration, but make sure the sound is coming from a place of relaxation. This section of the exercise will take three to five minutes.

Then start to gently rub your hands together, and place your palms on your eyes, letting your eyes drink in their warmth. Move your hands down your face, and rub your temples, then your scalp, drawing the head to one side as you massage the other. Rub the top of your head, then the forehead, cheeks, and jaw. You may even reach into the inside of your lips and cheeks and gently massage your inner cheeks (by pinching inside and outside with your thumb and index fingers). Then make soft upward strokes from your throat to your sternum to below your jaw. This position of the sequence will take about five minutes.

Place your index fingers under your lower earlobes at your upper jaw, and press in. Next, take your index fingers into the points above your collarbones alongside your neck, and rub from the center to the edges of your shoulders. Take your shoulders from underneath your upper back and rub as much and as hard as you like. Then take all four fingertips to the center of your chest and sweep your way out from the center. You can do this horizontally, and continue down your chest two inches at a time, repeating the sweeping from the center to the outside parameter of your chest. Finally, place your hands back over your heart (left under right) and move your hands in a circle from left to right over the Anahata Chakra   the heart center in the middle of the chest. Let yourself rest and absorb this delicious experience.

Follow with a heart-opening meditation if you like (see Chapter Seven).

Using Props for Self-Massage

It can be useful to use props when administering self-massage. Since you don't have another person to apply pressure, using an object and gravity will help to pinpoint and deepen the work. A rubber ball or foam cylinder or half cylinder can be very helpful for releasing tension from the muscles and fascia (connective tissue). Using your weight in combination with the object you are resting on will help you to apply gravity and pressure on the areas you are working. For instance, you can take a foam half cylinder and perch your outer thigh on the object (while resting some weight on your hands and forearms), then try rolling up and down the length of your outer leg. Then try a rubber ball under your shoulder blade: lie down, knees bent, and roll your shoulder weight from the lower to the upper point on the muscle and tendon. Go slowly and pause if you find points that feel like they need pressure. Breathe. Be creative and follow your instincts when using the props. It's a good idea to have a yoga block or two and a few blankets handy for practice.

chapter five

The Breathing Exercises

Breath is contact with life. From the minute we are born, we breathe. Nourishing our breath literally expands our quality of life. Through the practice of pranayama, or breath control, we are capable of prolonging mental, physical, and emotional well-being. By expanding our capacity to breathe, we are literally expanding our capacity to live. And, from a beauty standpoint, breathwork is an invaluable tool for bringing youth and vitality to all our facial features.

Increased oxygen levels translate as increased vitality to the skin, relieving symptoms of pallor, countering sagginess, and aiding in the healing process, as well as rallying white blood cell count to areas of infection more promptly. The muscles crave oxygen to function maximally, and deeper breathing will naturally assist the facial muscles in maintaining suppleness and a more firm resiliency. Deep breathing sends signals to the nervous system to relax and let go, which tells the skin to release facial expressions such as fear, worry, anger, and gripping, which age the face.

Deep breathing counters the fight-or-flight response by soothing the sympathetic nervous system. These days we are more threatened by ephemeral, mental constructs and presuppositions than by a natural force such as a woolly mammoth charging our way, but when the sympathetic nervous system feels threatened, it is hardwired to go into defense mode by producing higher levels of adrenaline, epinephrine, and norepinephrine, as well as releasing nutrients that cause muscular action (which can be toxic in the body when not needed), and inhibiting the digestive system (the cramp in the stomach produced by fear). All of this is hard on the body and accelerates the aging process.

The fight-or-flight response also inhibits the function of the tear glands and salivation, causing dehydration, and dilates the pupils and blood vessels. In the short run, the stress produced by the body's accelerating to the fight-or-flight response causes your skin to pale and your hairs to "stand on end," but in the long run, protracted episodes can lead to more long-term health problems, all of which are associated with the aging process.

The facial muscles respond to fear and stress by clutching, gripping, and assuming the "mask of fear." These expressions will etch themselves on the face after repeated involuntary responses, until they become the "signature expression." Think of grotesque symbols such as the joker or the dramatic emblems of tragedy and comedy— as we age, our repeated emotional responses are ingrained upon our faces. We literally carve our own facial masks through repeated emotional responses.

Deep breathing slows down the heart rate, sends oxygen to the circulatory system, and relaxes the nervous system to prevent the fight-or-flight response from taking over and running rampant. In other words, deep breathing will stop premature aging by stopping the fight-or-flight response in its tracks.

Wouldn't you rather have your habitual expressions be like the unfurrowed, sage-like neutrality of a Buddhist monk or the sweet and compassionate softness of a loving mother than the anxious, threatening wrinkled face of someone who perceives a threat at every corner?

In yogic tradition, the science of breath control is considered to be highly powerful and is reserved for study with an experienced teacher. Certain health conditions are contraindicated in practicing pranayama, and you should consult with a doctor to ascertain whether these exercises are appropriate for you. The breath exercises I outline in this chapter, however, are simple and safe, and if you practice them consistently, you should begin to experience immediate results in the form of more radiant, glowing, and unwrinkled skin.

Diaphragmatic Breathing

The most important aspect of controlling breath is using your diaphragm. Most people do not breathe from the diaphragm at all, but rather through the chest. This deprives the lower lobes of the lungs of their full share of oxygen and prevents a healthy exchange of the respiratory gases.

Diaphragmatic breathing also increases the suction pressure in the thoracic cavity, improving the venous return of blood and reducing the load on the heart while enhancing circulatory function.

If you want to observe diaphragmatic breathing in action, check out a sleeping child or dog. Animals and children are masters of diaphragmatic breathing. So from watching them, we can infer that our natural state is one of calm as well.

Lie down on a yoga mat with one hand on the center of your chest and one below the rib cage. As you inhale, observe the lower part of the rib cage expanding and the ab-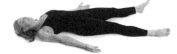
domen rising, and as you exhale, observe the opposite. The bulk of the movement should be occurring below the chest. You can also practice this breath in Savasana, or Corpse Pose, with your legs hip-width apart, palms up, and shoulders releasing down your

back on the floor. Couple this with a soft rolled-up blanket under your knees, and perhaps an eye pillow, to maximize your relaxation. Do this for two to three minutes.

You can also practice diaphragmatic breathing while standing, legs about hip-width apart, knees unlocked, and one hand on the lower abdomen. Simply direct your breath down to your belly and feel your hand rise and fall.

Try simply pausing at any point in the day to check where your breath is expanding and contracting. If you find your breathing is shallow and your belly isn't moving, take a conscious, belly-expanding breath. Place a hand on your belly to make sure you are directing your breath correctly. If you sit at a desk, sit in an upright position in your chair and keep your eyes level to whatever you are watching (most likely your computer). Do not slump back in your chair, and consider using an ergonomic pillow that supports an easy upright seat if you are at the desk all day. This way, you will keep your spine healthy, which will allow for deeper breathing.

Ironically, many people—especially women—are afraid of diaphragmatic breathing at first, because it encourages releasing the belly. But don't be afraid to round your belly. When I am teaching, I always urge my students to let their bellies grow fat with breath. If you take a moment to expand your belly with breath, chances are you won't feel the need to do it permanently with overeating. By the same token, inhaling deeply from a cigarette is an attempt to reproduce the relaxation that is created by a deep inhale—so a drag on a cigarette is really a roundabout way to breathe deeply. In taking a deep breath, we afford ourselves the opportunity to experience the truth in the moment. And practicing awareness of diaphragmatic breathing should help to cultivate it in your daily life.

Kapalabhati Breathing

Practicing Kapalabhati Breathing, or "skull shining breath," is a marvelous way to expel staleness and tiredness from the system and to impart a glow to the face, as the name suggests. It cleans the sinuses and respiratory system and tones the abdominals and digestive system. It is a form of diaphragmatic pumping that pushes oxygen up and clears stale air from the lungs. The diaphragm muscle actually massages the base of the heart when the pumping is performed strongly. The focus is on the exhale, and it involves a series of short, sharp exhaled bursts through the nose, followed by an immediate, shorter inhale. (One of my teachers, Peter Rizzo, calls it a rapid-fire nose-blowing session—have tissues handy!) Kaphalabhati Breathing increases circulation and purges toxins, and is extremely invigorating and cleansing.

Sit in Sukhasana (cross-legged seated position). Plant the sit bones and lengthen the spine. Broaden your collarbones and allow your shoulder blades to descend toward the waist. Place your hands, palms up, on your knees. Take a deep inhale through your nose down to the pelvic floor. Expel all the breath out in one deep exhale. Inhale to a comfortable level, and begin: Exhale sharply through the nose, follow with an involuntary intake of breath, and repeat for sixteen counts.

Then exhale out *all the breath* on the sixteenth exhalation, emptying the breath, and engage Mulabandha (root lock) by contracting the muscles and lifting the region between the anus and the genitals. Then apply Uddiyana Bandha by drawing the region two inches below the navel in and up. Now, with the two root locks applied, breathe a comfortable breath to the upper chamber of the chest, letting it rise like a balloon, and cap this breath by tucking your chin toward your sternum (the neck lock, Jalandhara Bandha). This breath retention—or kumbhaka—is highly powerful and should be held without gripping or aggressively clamping. It is said that this practice helps to create a less reactive mind. You are redirecting your prana—or life force—to the upper chamber of your chest, thereby reversing the downward flow of energy. Once you have tried this with sixteen counts, you can increase the number to forty or sixty. This breath technique is excellent to revive flagging energy.

Nauli Kriya

A kriya is a form of cleansing. The Nauli Kriya tones the abdominals and cleanses the digestive system.

Stand with your feet hip-width apart and your knees slightly soft. On an inhale, arch your back and exhale to a modified standing squat. After emptying the breath out through your mouth, stick out your buttocks, hollow your belly, round your back, tuck your chin to the hollow of your throat, and apply Uddiyana Bandha. Ripple the abdominal muscles from the base of your pubic bone up to the navel, several times in a row without taking in breath, like a belly dancer undulating her stomach. Never force the abdominal muscles outward; focus on the inward motion. When you run out of breath, roll up, with your chin to your chest, knees bent, and your head coming up last. Inhale and arch your back, repeat twice.

This exercise is always a hit in Yoga Face classes—it immediately gives you a highly oxygenated, rosy and radiant complexion. You will be filled with energy, and your body temperature will increase a bit. You may feel tingly or a little dizzy, as this exercise really moves and unblocks energy.

Note: do *not* do this exercise on a full stomach or if you have high blood pressure, a hiatal hernia, or heart disorder, or if you are pregnant or menstruating.

Alternate Nostril Breathing (Anuloma Viloma)

This is one of the main pranayama techniques, and it is helpful on many levels. In terms of facial beauty, it will prevent your nose from drooping as you age, and it will sculpt, firm, and define your nose. It helps to equalize your two major energy systems—the sun and moon channels. We often breathe more dominantly through one nostril, creating an imbalance. This breathing technique brings the breath back in evenly. Breathing predominantly through the left side indicates a creative, receptive mind-set, while breathing through the right produces a more regimented, "get it done" mind-set.

Sit comfortably in Sukhasana (cross-legged seated position). Take the first two fingers of your right hand to your right palm. Let your left hand sit palm-up on your left thigh or knee with your thumb and middle finger touching. You'll be using the thumb and ring finger of your right hand to regulate your breath flow, alternately through the left and right nostrils. Close your right nostril with your right thumb, inhale, then exhale out a slow, steady breath through your left nostril until the breath is spent.

At the bottom of the exhale, close your left nostril with your ring finger and open your right nostril. Inhale smoothly and completely. Repeat, inhaling through the left and exhaling through the right side twice. At the end of the third inhalation in the right nostril, exhale through the same side. Then close the right nostril and breathe through the left. Repeat this twice for a total of three sequences on each side. When you get more comfortable with this breathing, try doing alternate nostril breathing without holding your nostrils down as you regulate left to right (look, Ma, no hands!). This is considered to be a more advanced and pure form of the practice and will refine the contours of your nose.

Alternate nostril breathing is calming and is excellent at any time of the day or evening.

Ujjayi Breath

Ujjayi breath comes from the Sanskrit root *jai*, meaning victory. Ujjayi is the practice of deep, audible, partially restricted nasal breath (the folds in the back of the throat, or glottals, are restricted). It is thought that Ujjayi breath is purer and goes deeper to the circulatory and respiratory system. Nasal breathing is considered to be purer than mouth breathing, as the mucous membranes in the nose act as filters. During asana practice, Ujjayi breath helps the mind stay focused and the body receive deeper levels of oxygen, which in turn nourishes the blood, tissues, nerves, and muscles, producing calm, strength, and flexibility. The face receives better circulation as well and will appear more luminous and rosier. Breathe in through your nose, directing the breath up to the upper palate, and then send it to the back of your throat so it makes a whispering sound. As you exhale, let the breath hit the top of the back of your throat and upper palate so you can still hear it. (It sounds a little like Darth Vader's breathing—he was an advanced Jedi Knight, after all!) Listening to this breath as you meditate or do your asana practice is a way to direct your concentration.

Breath of Fire (Agni Prana)

This type of breathing is beneficial for generating heat, as its name suggests. Use this breathing technique when sitting in Sukhasana or when holding a pose—such as tabletop pose or incline plank to kick it up a notch. To do breath of fire, take rapid diaphragmatic breaths of even duration through your nose. Make the breaths swift and frequent—more than one breath per second. The emphasis is on the inhale; the exhale is passive. This breath may cause perspiration and light-headedness, but it is not hyperventilation. The sound of breath of fire has always reminded me of a hyena snickering, or at least what I imagine it would sound like.

The benefits of breath of fire include stress reduction, increased energy and endurance, cessation of addictive impulses, release of toxins from the mucous membranes of the lungs, balancing of the sympathetic and parasympathetic nervous systems, and nerve stimulation, and increased production of epinephrine and norepenephrine (the "feel good" brain chemicals that create a sense of optimism and regulate the appetite). The face will be radiant, glowing, and smooth.

· · ·

The cultivation of mindful breathing is a cornerstone of yoga practice, and is also an indispensable tool for enhancing youth, beauty, and overall quality of life. The beauty of breathwork is that it is relatively easy to perform, and it gives you incredibly beneficial results in a short time. No matter how pressed we are for time or how urgent things seem, it is always possible to slow down and practice mindful breathing techniques. To keep it really simple, pay attention to your breath and its rhythm at any given moment during the day. This will help you stay calm, present, and grounded. The breath practices are rightly considered by yogis to be more valuable than gold: they are sacred keys to unlocking vitality and preserving youth.

chapter six

Opening the Voice

Hare Rama, Hare Rama, Rama Rama, Hare Hare. Hare Krishna, Krishna Krishna, Krishna Krishna, Hare Hare . . . " The strains of kirtan, or communal singing as spiritual practice, rippled through my spine. It was in the middle of a humid New York City summer, in the old Jivamukti Yoga Center on Second Avenue in Manhattan. The much-beloved and highly touted Krishna Das, a sort of yogic Tom Waits (by way of Brooklyn) played the harmonium (a yogic accordion/keyboard) and led the Indian musicians, as well as about two hundred people, in the chant.

The candlelight danced, and as I looked around with a huge smile on my face, I saw arms outstretched, bodies swaying, and lots of sweet, beaming faces. As the scent of incense wafted through the air, a devotee walked around the room, reverentially giving us prasad, the blessed dessert symbolic of divine grace. We sang together, sometimes quietly, sometimes almost bellowing, and gradually opened up to our voices and each other. It was a diverse crowd: every color of skin and age from eighteen to eighty was represented, along with different economic backgrounds, professions, and faiths.

We all had one thing in common at that moment: our faces were beaming and completely youthful. We were full of joy and had let go of tension. It had been a while since I had sung in public, and I had never done so easily or unself-consciously, but now, at Jivamukti, I started to cry. Not from sadness, but from a sharp, joyous expansion of my heart.

When was the last time I had sung fully and expressively? It seemed like I never really had. Although I had been trained as a performer and had actually sung on stage, I had never before felt so vocally or emotionally free in my singing. Perhaps it was because this time I wasn't "performing" at all—I was experiencing the freedom of singing for joy. When I left the center and poured back into the busy East Village streets, people smiled at me spontaneously. I couldn't figure out what they were smiling at until I accidentally caught my reflection in a St. Mark's Place street vendor's mirror: I was smiling, no, grinning, from ear to ear. This smile probably had been plastered on my face for hours. I had no idea.

That night ushered in a joyous phase of deep devotion to my yoga practice—and I began to see the results on my face immediately. I started getting carded at nightclubs, even though I was in my thirties. I hadn't even been asked for ID when I was an underage, precocious teen. But now I looked younger at thirty-three than I ever had before. Once in a while I would run into a friend or acquaintance, and they'd inevitably ask, "What have you been doing? You look great!" They were stunned when I told them I hadn't been to a spa or gone on vacation, I was just attending kirtan sessions. The freedom I felt that night brought me back again and again; even years of vocal training hadn't given me what I got in that kirtan.

When was the last time you had a good singing session? How about singing in public? When was the last time you really raised your voice? And what were you feeling at the time? Perhaps it was when you were driving and someone cut you off? The car is one of the rare places where we can indulge in vocal self-expression in modern society because no one can hear us.

For most of us, full-out vocalization is rare, reserved for peak moments of emotion, such as anger, great fear, or unmitigated joy. We as a society are becoming decidedly less verbally expressive, and many of us will spend entire days in front of a computer typing on a keyboard for expression rather than using our mouths. It's almost as if our mouths have become flabby appendages, more for decoration than self-expression.

And yet the sheer, organic joy of spoken or sung self-expression is not only a delight; we humans are hardwired to produce sound and communicate vocally. On a primal level, we still need to discharge emotion and thoughts, and when we repress them, we bear the brunt in our faces and bodies. Locked jaws, slumped shoulders, burning acid stomachs, clenched fists, and tightened buttocks are all symptoms of unexpressed emotion. Scowls and marionette lines emerge on the face as a result of these tamped-down emotions. Eventually, habitual repression of emotions and thoughts shows up on our face in the form of wrinkles. In my work teaching the Yoga Face, I have seen people drop ten years in facial appearance in one hour, just from releasing unexpressed tension.

But what exactly happens when we vocalize? The production of sound involves a coordinated team of players: the lips, teeth, tongue, jaw, larynx (voice box), vocal chords, esophagus (windpipe), diaphragm, and lungs. The impulse to speak arises in your brain, leading to an intake of breath in the diaphragm and then the lungs, which is then released back out as an exhalation that travels through the windpipe and the mouth, resonating off the bones of the face and skull, and leading to a word, exclamation, or a sung note.

What is interesting and unique about vocalization is that emotion is so deeply connected to making sound: the impetus to communicate is not purely a physical need directly related to survival; it is also highly emotional. The less time the brain has to intermediate the impulsive sound (as in to judge or critique), the better and clearer the sound usually is.

Being unable to express ourselves vocally is not only deeply frustrating; it can be toxic. The English language is full of expressions that vividly describe this: "biting my tongue," "swallowing my pride," "grin and bear it." It is both interesting and a little sad to me that the once common practice of singing is on the wane. As technology has grown more sophisticated, people don't gather together to entertain themselves with stories and songs like they used to. I believe that this loss of communal self-expression has led to a decline in both physical and emotional health.

Singing is a marvelous way to express emotion. In some cultures, singing is still an integral part of socializing. The Japanese have a strong connection to singing as a group ritual. It is no surprise that they were the ones who invented karaoke, and it isn't uncommon in Japan to have a company or school song that people sing together often. In many Latin American countries, singing at parties with the accompaniment of a guitar is common. Unfortunately, in the United States, we seem to have gotten rather shy about singing in public, though we are still drawn to the mysterious power of song, as witnessed by our cultural fascination with shows such as *American Idol*. Fewer people belong to church or school choirs, and the only time many of us actually sing in public as a society is at a sports stadium.

Yogic philosophy recognizes that there are different pathways to realization, or enlightenment. One of these paths of yoga is the path of bhakti, or devotion: bhakti yogis chant and sing their way to realization. This vocalizing to a higher power is a venerated spiritual tradition, especially in southern India, where people may travel miles to attend kirtans. The path of bhakti is an ecstatic one, and attending a kirtan can be a transcendental experience. The tradition has a parallel in the United States with gospel music.

So as you are doing these vocalizing and singing exercises, be aware of the way they play upon your spirit, mood, and heart, and how they massage and release your vocal chords and facial muscles. Just opening up to the vibrations of this strong practice will shift your energy and your appearance.

Picking Grapes

Stand comfortably, arms at your side, feet hip-width apart, knees unlocked. Inhale through your nose and reach arms your up to the ceiling, hold the breath, and then "pick grapes" by reaching up alternate arms and inhaling a little more air each time. Do this until you can't take in anymore breathe. Then on the exhale, arch your back, swing your arms down, bend your knees, and go into a forward bend. Repeat three or four times. This exercise helps you stretch your intercostal muscles so you can expand your breathing apparatus, taking in more breath and allowing for powerful sound. It also will bring a lot of oxygen to your face.

The Om Sound

Lie down on a mat in Reclining Goddess Pose, with the soles of your feet together and your knees apart. Put some padding under your knees if they are tight. Place your hands on your abdomen and open your mouth wide. Let your lower jaw hang open and drop your tongue to the floor of your jaw. Say *aaaaah*.

Now place your hands on your heart and say *ooooh*, rounding your lips and feeling the vibrational quality of the sound.

Next place your hands on the sides of your head and chant *mmmmm*. Attune yourself to the vibrational quality of the *mmmmm* sound. Feel where in the body you are experiencing the vibration.

Now chant the three sound together: *aaaaah-ooooo-mmmmm*. Loop the sound until you aren't sure where it begins and where it ends. Keep your mouth open as wide as possible, but stay relaxed and don't jut out your head. The *om* sound is a tuning bell for your emotional, mental, physical, and spiritual health.

You can also do this exercise sitting on a cushion in a cross-legged seated position, either after doing it lying down or instead of it. Making sounds while lying down is great for eliminating tension and it allows you to connect to your breathing.

Voicing Vowels While Lying Down

Lie down with your knees bent and your feet on the floor. Relax and let your breath come in and out naturally. Place one hand on your lower abdomen and feel the breath rise and fall. Then imagine your "highway of sound": a large tunnel or tube that starts at the crown of your head and travels unimpeded through your windpipe, esophagus, diaphragm, and into the pelvic floor two inches below your navel. Let the impulse for sound drop as breath through the crown of your head or the nose and mouth (whichever feels more organic to you), travel to the pelvic floor, and release as a soft *shhhhh*.

Repeat this exercise for three to five minutes. Do not force the sound; let it drop in naturally and then release with *shhhhh*. Next, begin to let yourself receive breath as sound, and exhale on the sound *hu-hum*. Let the *hu-hum* sound come from your diaphragm. Again, let the impulse for sound drop in through the crown of your head to the pelvic floor, then release on a soft diaphragmatic *hu-hummmm-mmmm*. Do not force this sound. It should feel like a hiccup, but deeper. Practice *hu-hum* for two minutes.

Next, try *aaaaah*. Let your lips drop to the floor of your jaw, and let the jaw relax. Let the breath drop in as sound, drop through your pelvic floor, and release through your mouth as *oooooh*. Repeat this several times, then use the *eeeee* sound, then the *iiiii* sound. Go through the vowels. Don't force the sounds; let yourself be in a state of receptive relaxation. Notice the different color and vibrational quality of each different vowel sound. Do they come from different parts of your body? Do you prefer one vowel sound to another? Picture each vowel with a particular color.

Mini Vowel Exercise for Facial Toning

You can shorten the vowel sound exercise for a pure facial workout by looking in the mirror and saying all the vowel sounds and exaggerating the lip and mouth movements to *really enunciate*. Repeat five times to tone the cheeks, lips, and jaw.

Consonants

Consonants are a different experience, both in sound production and in emotional quality. They are naturally harder and more sharp, and often more forceful. Use them to express yourself—especially more energetic emotions, such as passion or anger—and to work out your mouth and the rest of your vocal apparatus.

Lie down, knees bent, with one hand on your belly, and allow sound to drop in through the crown of your head and down your "highway of sound" as breath and leave your body as a voiced consonant. Go through the alphabet from start to finish, one consonant at a time. Do not say the name of each letter, but rather, make the consonant sound. (For example, for *b, c, d, f*, vocalize crisply and sharply, *buh, sss, duh, ffff*.) Again, let the different shades of color and mood wash through you with each consonant and see which feel easier to express and are more satisfying.

Chanting

Chanting in Sanskrit is very good for the voice. Since Sanskrit is a vibrational language, it lends itself to easy sound production and will warm up and enrich your voice. Rather than singing scales, try singing a chant as a scale (like do-re-mi), starting low and going higher with each repetition. Keep your mouth open and your tongue dropping to the floor of your jaw. Don't jut your neck out, as it will cause tension and inhibit sound. Keep your knees loose. You may get quite warm singing. In the pages that follow, I offer a range of chants to choose from. After a good ten to twenty minutes of chanting, you may follow with meditation—this energizing practice will help you focus. Then look at your face. You may be truly shocked at the transformation. Enjoy!

(A note on Sanskrit: you can be of any faith—including none—and derive benefit from chanting these words. Although they are not religious, they are spiritual, and are all-encompassing. Yoga is not considered to be a religion, but a philosophy and science.)

The Seed Mantras: A Sound Meditation

In yogic philosophy, the chakras are spinning wheels of energy that are situated on the main energy pathways of the body. The seven main chakras are located on the spinal column, the first, or root chakra, is at the base of the spine. The second is under the navel. The third is at the region of the solar plexus. The fourth chakra is at the heart center. The fifth is at the throat, and the sixth is at the point between the eyebrows (the third eye). The last chakra at the crown of the head is called the thousand-petaled lotus and is considered to be evolutionarily the highest. In yogic philosophy, this last chakra is considered the pathway to divine consciousness.

Each chakra has a bija, or seed, mantra, or root sound, and chanting these sounds is a wonderful way of connecting with your power, vitality, and creativity as well as letting go of the tensions of the day to feel more calm and peaceful.

Take an easy cross-legged seated position. You may sit on some padding to make yourself more comfortable. Place your hands on your knees, palms up, and press your index fingers to your thumbs.

You will chant the sound of each chakra from the base of your spine up to the crown. Open your mouth widely as you chant and release your tongue. Do not strain your neck; keep your head poised elegantly on top of your spine. Experience the vibratory quality of the sound as it resonates through your body. You don't need to visualize the chakras, but you can do so if you like. I like to connect to the sound itself as I chant and let the power of the mantra take hold. This is an entire chakra sound meditation, but if you want to concentrate on opening up a specific center, you can choose to chant just the one sound of that specific chakra. For instance, if you want to feel more grounded and stable at any time in the day, chant the seed sound for the first chakra, *lam*. If you want to feel more creative, chant *vam*. If you want to improve your self-confidence, chant *ram*.

1. Root (Muladhara) Chakra

The root chakra, located at the base of the spine, is the seat of survival, earth, obtaining, and saving resources. It correlates with physical identity, the bones, energy pathways, and the hair. The corresponding color is yellow. Kundalini, the sacred force of existence and enlightenment, represented by a serpent, is situated here.

This chakra is associated with the skin, so chanting its bija mantra, *lam*, will help give you healthier, more glowing skin.

Chant *lam* seven times. Pause. Repeat once.

2. Sacral (Swadhisthana) Chakra

The second chakra is the center of sexuality, creativity, and the sense of taste. The element is water. It is located about two fingers below the navel, and is the "feel good" center. Connection to the second chakra brings a sense of fluidity and grace, and a feeling of attractiveness and is associated with regulating sex hormones. Chant its bija mantra, *vam*, to feel sexually, creatively, and interpersonally aligned.

Chant *vam* seven times. Repeat once.

3. Navel (Manipura) Chakra

The third chakra, located behind the navel, at the solar plexus, is associated with personal power and egoic force. Its element is fire. Confidence, discipline, and self-esteem can be obtained from chanting its bija mantra, *ram*. Metabolism is governed from this chakra.

Chant *ram* seven times, pause, and repeat once.

4. Heart (Anahata) Chakra

The fourth chakra is the first chakra of transcending individual ego. Its element is air. Located in the center of the chest, this center is where love and compassion emanate. The heart, arms, hands, and legs all are linked to this center. To feel loved and to love more freely, connect with this center by chanting its bija mantra, *yam*.

Chant *yam* seven times, pause, and repeat once.

5. Throat (Vishuddha) Chakra

The fifth chakra is associated with self-expression and creative voice. The throat and mouth are governed by this center, so chant the bija mantra to increase health and attractiveness in these regions. The element here is sound. Chant its mantra, *ham*, to clear out communication or self-assertion blocks and to give voice to your truth.

Chant *ham* seven times, pause, and repeat once.

6. Third-Eye (Ajana) Chakra

The sixth chakra, located between the eyebrows, is considered to be the seat of the highest self, and also the center for intuition and divine interface. To see clearly, to hone intuition, and to feel connected to your highest inner teacher, chant its bija mantra, *om*. The sixth chakra is associated with the pineal gland, which regulates aging. It is thought that in the aging process, calcification prohibits healthy regulation of melatonin (the sleep hormone). Melatonin is also associated with immune function and "feeling good." As we age, many of us tend to lose sleep. Seventh chakra work will help regulate sleep function. It also governs sight and seeing.

Chant *om* seven times. Repeat once.

7. Crown (Sahashrara) Chakra

The seventh chakra, at the crown of the head, is the thousand-petaled lotus. It symbolizes connection to the universal divine force, and self-knowledge and spiritual consciousness. Chant its mantra, *om*.

Chant *om* seven times more. Repeat once. Sit and meditate on the *om* sound, five minutes or more.

The following chants are wonderful to do in the morning as a spoken affirmation or prayer. You can either pick one from the following list and chant it ten to twenty times, pick your own tune, or just chant in a spoken voice.

1. *Om namah shivaya* (I bow to my highest inner truth and teacher)
2. *Om shanti, om shanti, om shanti, om* (Peace, peace, peace)
3. *Loka samasta sukhino bhavantu* (May all beings everywhere be happy and free)
4. *Isvara pranavah* (I surrender to the divine)
5. *Yogas citta vritti nirodha* (Pronounced "yogash cheetah vreetee neerodaha": yoga is the quieting of mind chatter)
6. In Latin: *Dona nobis pacem* (Give us peace)

Singing to Yourself

Sit in an easy cross-legged seated position and close your eyes. Relax and let your breath rise and fall. Sing a song. If you feel yourself tensing, notice it without judgment and let it go. Try singing a song that makes you feel devotional or happy. "Amazing Grace" is a good one. You may sing any prayer or poem you know or make one up. Try to express how you really feel. Make up your own tune. If you play an instrument, accompany yourself. If you don't play an instrument, you can lightly tap your hands on your lap or clap in time. Or pick up some finger bells or a small drum at your local music or Indian store. Let Sarasvati, the goddess of music, inspire you.

Try singing an affirmation:

I am happy
I am free
I am happy to be me
I am joyous, I'm divine
I'll be yours and you'll be mine

Or sing any other spiritual song that moves you.

You can try putting on recordings of songs you love to sing and singing along—or make up your own—try it when you are home alone, cleaning the house . . .

Singing and opening up the voice are keys to joy and self-expression. Children quite freely sing and voice their emotions, and their faces are clear and their eyes are shiny. Being able to express yourself fearlessly and joyfully will put you in touch with the energy of your heart, which has no age. Once you see and feel the results of these lovely practices, you will crave them more and more. Maybe you can invite people over for a singing or chanting party. Even just two people can make a mini-choir. Have fun!

chapter seven

It's All in Your Mind

People often say to me, "I would love to meditate, but I don't have the time." I have been known to use this excuse myself. But the truth is, even five minutes of meditation is time well spent—time that will help calm the mind and slow down the spinning world for a moment. By creating a little time to meditate, you are ultimately clearing the decks so that you can have a more blissful, energized focus. People who meditate consistently look more radiant, peaceful, and younger, the antithesis of a scowling, frowning worrywart. Also, people who meditate tend to have slower heart rates and lower stress levels. They report feeling calmer and more focused, and tend to be more positive. Do you really not have the time for this?

"Mind over matter."
"It's all in your mind."
"As the mind, so the man."

These are some of the phrases we use to say that whatever you focus on, you become. This is especially true in terms of your self-image. If you worry about getting older and losing your vitality, the worry tends to produce that very effect. Using your energy to take a positive action is the best antidote to this kind of worry. In fact, taking the time to relax your mind is one of the key components of the Yoga Face program, and it will help you drop years off your face. Letting go is instrumental in keeping a youthful appearance. It helps the facial muscles unclench and stop gripping in unattractive shapes. Think of it as one of the main facets of facial rejuvenation.

There are many different types of meditation. Because people are unique, a meditation that works for some may leave others cold. And you may go through different phases—at one point you may love just sitting and listening to your breath moving in and out, and at other times you may need something more active, like mantra repetition or a visualization exercise. Learning how to discipline and harness your mental energy is an invaluable tool, not only for looking years better, but for creating a positive mental state that facilitates envisioning and implementing the life you want to create.

Meditation and mental training can help you to take responsibility for your life. We all think constantly—thousands of thoughts a day. Many of these thoughts are so repetitive that we stop noticing them altogether. Meditation allows us to be still enough to watch the mind do its thing, without judgment, and to detach a little. Once we do this, we stop identifying with ego-based thoughts, and may be able to let go of unconscious, compulsive behaviors.

Meditation is a practice, and like other forms of practice, it isn't how much you achieve that matters so much as just showing up. So suit up and show up, be a little willing, and get ready to watch your face, mind, and the rest of your life change.

. . .

Find a place where you are able to sit comfortably, and if necessary give yourself support with padding under your knees, behind your back, or underneath the sit bones to help the hips and knees release a little. Once you have picked a steady, comfortable seat, do not fidget or shift unless absolutely necessary. (This does not mean you should be harsh on yourself. Once when I was on a retreat I sat in a half-lotus pose—for me, a pretty uncomfortable position—and refused to budge out of fear of displeasing my teacher. I ended up giving myself a knee problem that bothers me to this day.)

The following meditations can all be practiced anywhere from five to twenty minutes. Try to increase the duration of your meditations incrementally, starting at five minutes and gradually increasing your sitting periods by a minute or two. Consider this training for the mind, similar to an athlete inceasing endurance over time.

Candle Flame Meditation

This meditation is good for beginners because it is so concrete. It is an exercise in seeing and perception that works the orbicularis ring muscles around the eyes, fighting crow's-feet and other eye wrinkles.

Take a candle and place it at eye level, either in an easy seated pose cross-legged on a cushion or sitting comfortably in a chair. Light the candle and look at the flame. Try to absorb every detail with your eyes. When you have taken in as much information about the flame as possible, close your eyes and try to re-create in your mind's eye as accurately as possible what you observed. Then open your eyes and get a "reality check": notice how accurate your perception was, and absorb any new information that comes up. Then close your eyes again and re-create this newly updated image. Go back and forth like this, beginning to incorporate more detail every time you open your eyes. You can start to absorb other parts of the candle as you go—the body of the candle itself, its holder, and so on. Do this for a minimum of five minutes, and try to work up to ten or even twenty minutes.

This meditation is great for developing concentration. It is dhyana meditation, one in which you focus on something outside yourself and begin to quiet the mind and become one with what you perceive. This is a way of gaining true understanding and yogic power. Because this meditation teaches light but steady visual focus and inner seeing, it will also help your eyes stay smooth and unwrinkled and your brow unfurrowed.

Flower Meditation

Follow the instructions for the Candle Flame Meditation, but substitute a flower for the candle. In fact, you can do this sort of meditation with any chosen object but obviously, beautiful and powerful objects are more appealing than ugly and disturbing ones.

Poem Meditation

Choose an uplifting passage from a poem you enjoy or a passage from a spiritual text that speaks to you. If you can't decide on one, open up a book you like and choose a random selection to meditate on. (I do this when I am feeling uninspired or simply want fate to intervene.) Then sit for five to twenty minutes contemplating the reading.

Meditation on Sound

Pick a sound that is constant in your environment—perhaps your own breath—and listen to it as closely as you can for five to ten minutes. Most likely your mind will chatter like a little monkey and find comments to fill the silence. It is your job to notice the thoughts without judgment, and to simply go back to concentrating on your sound.

You can also sit quietly with your eyes closed and listen to all the sounds that come up in your environment—without getting caught up in stories that your mind wishes to tell you about what you are observing. Obviously, a pleasant environment—such as a peaceful garden or a stretch of beach—is preferable to a jackhammer-infested city street for a listening meditation. You can also listen to a piece of uplifting or inspiring music. Again, if your mind begins to wander, notice it and pull it back like you would pull a child away from a distraction. Lying down during a music meditation can be very nice. Try to meditate for five to ten minutes.

Ocean Meditation

Sit by the ocean and listen to the waves. If you don't have the luxury of living near the beach, put on an audio recording of the ocean. (A jungle or a mountain stream recording will also work.) Try meditating on the ocean for five to ten minutes.

Mantra Meditation

Pick a word or phrase that resonates with you and repeat it silently in your mind. You may sing it in your mind as well. This is an effective meditation for people who are easily distracted (pretty much anyone living in modern society).

Here are some great mantras:

Om namah shivaya (I bow to my highest self)
Om mani padme om (I bow to the lotus blossom of enlightenment),
    or simply repeat *om* in your mind
Soham (I am that eternal truth)

If you prefer to repeat a prayer in English or another language, great! You may even pick a word that has resonance with you, like *peace* or *truth*. The advantage to mentally repeating Sanskrit is that most likely it is not your first language, so the meaning of the words will not distract you. Also, Sanskrit is considered to be a highly distilled, sacred, and powerful language: scholars refer to it as the mother of all languages. Its vibrational quality alone aids deep meditation.

Meditation on the Breath

There are many techniques for breath-centered meditation. Entire philosophies are founded upon breathing techniques. You may try any of these for between five and twenty minutes and see which works best for you.

Notice the in breath, notice the out breath.
Notice only the in breath.
Notice only the out breath.

Sama Vritti ("same breath"): Concentrate on making your inhale the same duration as your exhale. Count to four on the inhale, then count to four on the exhale. Do this for five to ten minutes. This is a highly effective method for stabilizing energy.

Third-Eye Meditation

Sit down in a comfortable position. Close your eyes and focus inwardly on the point between your eyebrows. This is your third-eye center and is considered to be the abode of Shiva, the highest self. Imagine a small disc of light or a pearl between your eyebrows. You may choose to fill this with a color such as white, blue, or silver.

Observe the disc pulsing and expanding, and try to let go of any agenda other than observing this point between the brows. Sit as long as you can—at least five minutes, or up to twenty or even thirty minutes. This meditation will help you tap into your intuition and your sense of truth.

Heart's Desire Visualization

Sit or lie down in a comfortable position. Imagine a guide—your own inner voice, or perhaps that of an ancestor or spiritual counselor. Or perhaps you feel inspired by a great teacher, such as Mother Teresa, Jesus, or Gandhi, whose actions you wish to emulate. Imagine this person coming to you and taking you on a path to your heart's desire. The more detailed you make the visualization the better. You can repeat the visualization several times, continuing to add more detail each time.

Imagine yourself walking through the forest, then reaching a bank of water or an ocean, and picture watching the water with your guide. Let your guide tell you what you need to do to attain your heart's desire.

Affirmations

Affirmations are very powerful. You may repeat them silently to yourself, in meditation, or throughout the day. You can also try looking at yourself in the mirror and repeating one or two of the following little gems to yourself. You may encounter some resistance; cultivating a peaceful and loving self-talk practice is difficult at first, especially if you are accustomed (as most of us are) to giving yourself negative messages.

At first when you repeat one of these positive affirmations, you might hear the judgmental voice inside your head respond with something negative. Simply smile and counter whatever protest the negative voice comes up with with another positive statement. Repeat the affirmation a few more times, varying your vocal patterns and the words you emphasize. Here are some you may try, or feel free to invent your own.

My face is sweet and smooth. I radiate health and am rejuvenated.

Breathing in, I smile to myself. Breathing out, I let go of tension.

As I live I grow.

I love to love and be loved.

I radiate goodness, I radiate joy.

I see beauty, I radiate beauty, I am beauty.

I receive joy and abundance with gratitude.

I am perfectly vibrant, strong, and healthy.

Here is an affirmation sequence that should be done in a seated position:

Breathing in, I breathe in light.
Breathing out, I release fear.
Breathing in, I breathe in joy.
Breathing out, I release despair.
Breathing in, I breathe in energy.
Breathing out, I let go of worry.
Breathing in, I am nourished.

Breathing out, I let go of clinging.

Breathing in, I am ageless.

Breathing out, tiredness leaves.

Breathing in, I am abundant.

Breathing out, I release what I don't need.

Praying for Others

In a comfortable seated position, visualize sending loving energy and healing to friends, family, and enemies, and then extend that energy to the entire world. You can imagine the loving healing energy coming from your heart in the form of a color (intuitively choose what feels like love to you), and then transmit the beams of the color onto the person, place, or thing you are blessing.

Blessing difficult people is a good way to translate a negative relationship into a positive one. We do not have to condone bad behavior to practice compassion. You may also endow the loving energetic color with a weight or shape—say a balloon of light that encompasses the person you are blessing.

Meditating with a Friend

Meditating with another person or a group is a wonderful way of enhancing concentration and doubling or even quadrupling the benefits of the practice. I find I am less prone to mentally wander when in the company of others focused on the same goal.

If you sit with one other person, face each other at a comfortable distance, and choose a meditation practice that suits you. If you are sitting with more than two people sit in a circle. You may start with a reading if you like, then set a timer for whatever period you wish. If you want to practice understanding and intimacy, try gazing into another person's eyes. See if you can maintain the other person's eyes as an object of meditation for thirty seconds to a minute. Perhaps you can build up to longer. Then try sitting and focusing on your own inner eye, with the outer eyes closed. You may wish to burn a candle during the meditation.

Transitional Visualization

Visualize yourself at different ages, and imagine your face at each age. Go chronologically. Try to remember yourself (even your idea of what you were like, or your intuitive sense of what you were like) at the age of one. Picture your face in your mind. Do the same for the age of three, then five, then seven, then ten, then fifteen, then twenty, then twenty-five, and so on, until you reach your current age.

With each mental picture of your face, spend time gazing into your own eyes and affirming this statement: I am ageless. I am eternal. I am the embodiment of life and joy.

Be patient and gentle with yourself as you practice these techniques. Over time, you undoubtedly will begin to drop the hard layers of self-protection that may keep you from relaxing your mind fully. You will experience more peace and health, and will receive the gift of a calmer, smoother face to boot.

In the next chapter, I will suggest some sequences in which you can combine the facial, vocal, and physical poses with the meditations and affirmations you have just discovered.

chapter eight

Sequences:
Putting It All Together

Think of this book as a collection of recipes. I have given you samples from several courses, and now it is time to feast on a meal. Part of what makes the Yoga Face program unique is that it draws upon a variety of techniques to help you rejuvenate your face. Rather than simply relying on a few facial stretches, yoga poses, or creams to do the trick, the Yoga Face takes a multitiered approach that works on different levels simultaneously. And, best of all, you can create your own personal program of exercises that work for you.

Creativity and improvisation are also important in the Yoga Face. Feel free to take from the different sections and choose the exercises that appeal to you. Chances are you intuitively will be drawn to the poses, stretches, meditations, and vocalizations that you need. Or you may want to work on the purely physical level first, and then incorporate the mind and relaxation exercises later on. You certainly have many choices and can mix things up as you progress. You may find that you respond to certain components of the book right away and will simply wish to continue practicing the same exercises for some time.

The more holistically you practice, though, the more benefits you will reap. I began to see my face changing through asana practice alone, but when I added facial poses, a new piece of the puzzle fell into place. Then I began adding the use of sound to the mix and really saw a difference. The mental component of meditation and affirmations brought not only release and openness to my facial features but also began to show up in my life as increased success, abundance, and prosperity. I found the mental component to be extremely powerful, for it affected every action I took, and it planted a seed of positivity in my mind that continues to bloom.

It is best to try to pick at least one exercise from each category every day. Because I wanted to give you a variety of options, I have included many exercises in this book, but by no means could anyone do them all every day. So in this chapter I have organized the sequences by thematic elements—water, air, earth, and fire—to help you practice in manageable pieces. At some point, you will want to add to or mix up your sequence or routine.

Each sequence includes at least one component of the individual categories of the Yoga Face (breathing practices, yoga poses, facial exercise, loving touch, meditation/affirmation, vocalization/chant).

The sequences build in physical intensity, with water being the most gentle, air a little more vigorous, earth more physical than air, and fire the most physically challenging. Each of these sequences will take you between twenty and forty minutes to complete, depending on your pace. Always feel free to modify or edit what doesn't work for you—remember, it's your body, and your practice. You may wish to select certain sections of these sequences to shorten the practice.

Play and have fun!

Water's essential qualities can change your mood, energy, and appearance. Water is receptive, so the exercises in this sequence are more about receiving energy and letting go. This sequence is restorative, meaning you will take in more energy than you will expend. It is a great practice for when you are tired and need restoration, and is also a wonderful tool for self-expression and the release of pent-up energies and emotions. It is ideal for a lazy weekend morning, or is a perfect practice to do an hour or so before bed, as it will help you to unwind and let go. If you practice before sleep, make sure you place a notepad or journal with a pen next to your bed to record your dreams upon awakening. Often you will receive valuable messages from your subconscious after this sequence. Because this practice will help you relax and feel more rested, your face will let go of tension and banish bloat, puffiness, and bags.

Breathing Practice

Alternate Nostril Breathing (*page 110*).

Yoga Poses

1. Lie down in Reclining Goddess Pose, with the soles of your feet together and your knees apart. Let your arms spread open, with your palms facing up. Feel your heart open, the blood pulsing in your body, and the weight of your body on the floor.

2. Let your breath be easy and natural. Do not practice any style; rather, allow your breath to move easily of its own accord. Stay here for three to five minutes.

3. Give yourself a face massage (*page* 93) for two or three minutes.

4. While lying in Goddess Pose, gently roll your head from side to side to loosen your neck. Now place your knees together, feet apart, and place your hands on your lower abdomen. Listen to your breath as you feel it rising and falling. Knock your bent knees off each other from side to side like windshield wipers five or six times. Then hug your knees toward your chest and rock your lower back in circles. Finally, rock and roll on your back with your knees to your chest, and rock up to sit.

5. From an easy cross-legged seat, inhale and raise your left arm toward the ceiling. Place your right fingertips, facing away from the seat, on the floor four inches behind your tailbone. Exhale, and place your left hand on the right knee. Inhale again to lengthen your spine, exhale to lightly deepen the twist. Inhale, lengthen your spine, exhale and look over your right shoulder. Now repeat this sequence in the opposite direction. Come to center and take the tip of your tongue behind your lower teeth, with your mouth open. Relax your tongue and jaw. Then stick out your tongue for as long as you can, keeping the rest of your face relaxed. Finally, circle your tongue around the perimeter of your mouth three or four times.

6. Relax your face and keep your teeth apart. Make sure your head is aligned on top of your spine, with your collarbones broad. Close your eyes and take your index fingers to the point right below your earlobes on the upper jaw, with your other fingertips and thumbs holding the jaw in place. Use your fingertips to rub the area in a spiraling motion, and continue this massage down the muscles and ligaments of the jaw, until you get to the hinge

point between the upper and lower jaws. Take your index and middle fingers to this hinge area, and rub as deeply as possible. As you do this massage, keep your face relaxed and exhale sound (such as *aaaaah*) to release tension. Do this for as long as you like—three minutes or so is a good amount of time. Then, after you have finished rubbing your jaw and exhaling out tension, tuck your chin toward your sternum and take your thumbs to the base of your skull alongside the top (atlas) vertebra, and rub at this pressure point.

In your cross-legged seated position, twist your arms, head, and torso to the right, then to the left, about thirty seconds in each direction. Bring your torso back to center and roll your head from shoulder to shoulder.

7. Lie down in Legs-Up-the-Wall Pose (*page 71*), a gentle inversion.

8. Fish Pose (*page 75*).

9. Corpse Pose (*page 65*) five to eight breaths for each.

10. Child's Pose (*page 58*). Rub the base of your skull and scalp in Child's Pose.

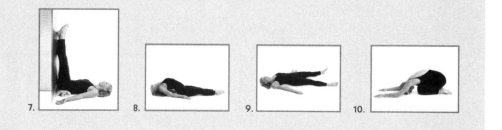

7. 8. 9. 10.

11. Cat/Cow (*page 77*) three to four times.

12. Downward-Facing Dog (*page 72*).

13. Walk to your feet and stand hanging over your legs, knees slightly bent. Clasp opposite elbows.

14. Roll up to standing.

15. Shrug your shoulders.

16. Cow Face Pose (*page 84*).

17. Standing Side Stretch (*page 86*).

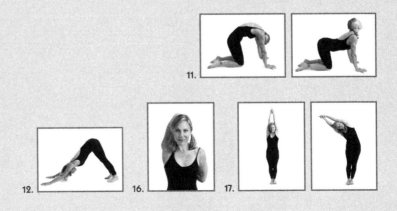

A quick reminder on the times of poses:

In general, a pose should be held for five to eight breaths, counting the inhale and the exhale as one unit of breath. However, this is not a firm mandate. You may wish to spend more time in poses that feel beneficial. The key is balance. Pay attention to the duration of your poses and your breathing. By paying close attention, you will be able to understand where you may have blocked energy.

Facial Exercises

Go to the mirror and do these facial exercises for the eyes and eyebrows:

1. Sphinx Smile (*page 17*).

2. Smiling Fish Face (*page 19*).

3. Temple Dancer Eyes (*page 32*).

4. Surprise Me! (*page 33*).

5. Brow Lift (*page 36*).

6. Crow, Crow, Go Away! (*page 35*).

7. Lion Face (*page 37*).

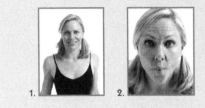

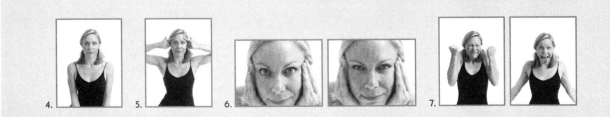

8. Gate Pose (*page 87*).

9. Child's Pose (*page 58*).

10. Star Pose (*page 60*).

11. Locust Pose (*page 79*).

12. Bridge Pose (*page 80*).

13. Legs-Up-the-Wall Pose (*page 71*).

14. Supine Twist (*page 84*).

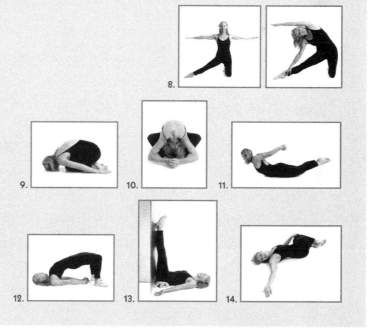

8.

9.   10.   11.

12.   13.   14.

Higher-Self Meditation

Choose a comfortable, easy seated position. Place your hands on your knees, palms up, elbows bent, shoulders released, and heart lifted. Close your eyes. Take your inner gaze to the point between the eyebrows, the symbolic seat of your highest self. Focus your mind on this point. Your mind will undoubtedly chatter with thought—this is, after all, the nature of the mind. Let thoughts wash through you, like birds on the wing flying through an empty temple—and return your inner gaze to the point between the brows. You may incorporate awareness of your breath into this meditation, but keep the primary focus on this point. Sit for a minimum of five minutes and up to twenty minutes.

Affirmation

After you have finished the meditation, silently repeat to yourself at least ten times, "I know the things I know."

Prayer

I pray for the ability to be receptive, like water. I pray that I may move through life without attachment, adjusting to my surroundings and joining the ocean of awareness like a drop in the sea.

Corpse Pose (page 65) to music (a gentle sound track such as mellow classical music or nature sounds).

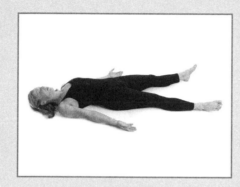

Come back to sitting.

Chant

Soham Soham (I am that eternal truth). Chant for five to ten minutes.

Enjoy the quiet, sweet, happy buzz of this practice and take a shower or bath afterward if you like. Rub some sweet oil on your skin, and smile.

Air moves swiftly, and in yoga is often linked with the intellect. Air is a wonderful element to use when "sweeping away" clutter and old habits. Let this practice blow away cobwebs and dust from your consciousness. The air sequence focuses on breathing (pranayama) techniques. Many advanced yogis believe pranayama practice is deeper than asana, since pranayama works directly with the life force. Because of this, you will notice the effects very quickly. This sequence will sweep away puffiness and bloating in your skin and take away heaviness from your facial features.

Easy Pose

Chant *om* three times.

Breathing Practice

Sama Vritti (page 132). Sama Vritti is a pranayama technique used to stabilize energy (*sama* comes from the Sanskrit for "same"). Simply put, make your inhale as long as your exhale by counting the incoming breath and matching the outgoing breath to it. I suggest a slow four count. Do this for three to five minutes.

Yoga Poses

1. Kundalini Spinal Propeller: This exercise stimulates kundalini energy. While seated, place your hands palms-down on your knees. Inhale, extend and roll your spine down over your right knee. Roll your spine back, still holding your knees down with your palms, and

exhale over your left knee as you round your spine. Repeat this counterclockwise motion three times, extending your arms as much as possible and lengthening your spine as you go. Now reverse the breath, inhaling over your left knee and exhaling over your right knee. Repeat three times, then come back to center.

2. Child's Pose (*page 58*) five breaths.

3. Threading the Needle (*page 59*) five breaths each side.

4. Cat/Cow (*page 77*) three times in a row.

5. Downward-Facing Dog (*page 72*), walk to your hands and roll up to stand for five counts.

6. Reach up to the heavens for energy, then make fists as you fold forward, and swing your arms back behind you. Repeat three times.

7. Circle your arms like windmills for about forty-five seconds.

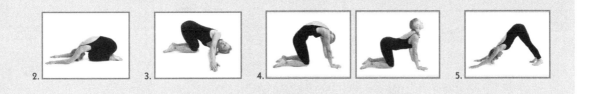

8. Swaying Tree (*page 99*): stand with your feet hip-width apart, knees unlocked. Make fists and swing your arms and trunk from side to side, allowing your fists to hit your buttocks and front leg oppositionally. Do this for thirty seconds.

9. Standing Side Stretch (*page 86*).

10. Mountain Pose (*page 50*).

11. Nauli Kriya (*page 110*).

12. From an easy cross-legged seat, do Head and Neck Rolls (*page 29*).

13. Seated Spinal Twists (*page 83*).

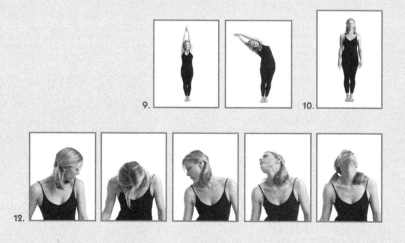

Facial Exercises

1. Free Your Tongue (*page 20*).

2. Tongue Tracing (*page 18*).

3. Bumblebees (*page 24*).

4. Marilyn (*page 16*).

5. Smiling Fish Face (*page 19*).

6. Chew sound, Bumblebees (*page 24*).

7. Lower Jaw Grip and Shake (*page 28*).

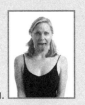

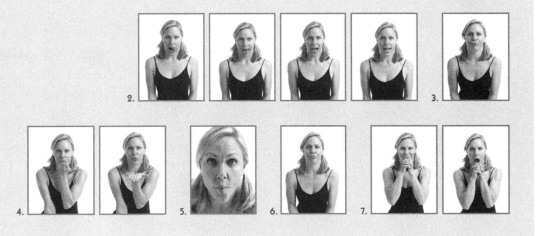

8. Jaw Release (*page 94*).

9. Yawn at least three times.

10. Seated Forward Bend (*page 60*).

11. Child's Pose (*page 58*).

12. Corpse Pose (*page 65*).

13. Plow Pose (*page 67*).

14. Shoulderstand (*page 69*) or Legs-Up-the-Wall Pose (*page 71*).

15. Fish Pose (*page 75*).

10.

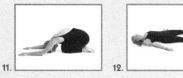

11.   12.

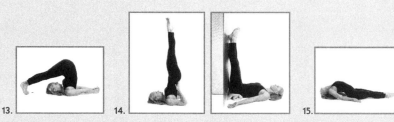

13.   14.   15.

Meditation

Listen to the in breath, listen to the out breath, for five minutes.

Chant

Chant *ham* (the throat center mantra) ten times for clear self-expression and vocal power. Do this for five minutes.

Prayer

I offer myself and my practice to the forces of air and wind, that old thoughts and patterns may be swept away, clearing space for the new.

Affirmation

I think clearly, I express myself clearly.

Rest in Corpse Pose (*page 65*).

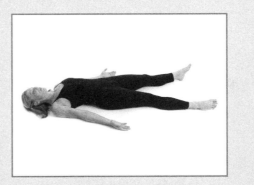

The earth sequence will give you a sense of beeing solid and grounded. Practice this sequence when you want to feel especially connected and healthy. It will help counter nervousness, illness, and anxiety, put you in touch with your internal power, and help you to create more stability and balance. Practice this sequence and get ready to make your mark and achieve prosperity. You will be less likely to be influenced by external events and faces. The following sequence will also improve your skin, teeth, and hair.

Chant

In Corpse Pose (page 65), chant *lam* eight times.

Breathing Practice

Kapalabhati (*page 108*)—then exhale all the breath, retain the breath, and apply Mulabandha, Uddiyana Bandha, and Jalandhara Bandha, and hold for as long as you comfortably can. When you need to, lift your chin and slowly exhale out through your nose. Inhale a new breath slowly. Do this for five minutes.

Yoga Poses

1. Mountain Pose (*page 50*).

2. Tree Pose (*page 54*).

3. Warrior 2 (*page 51*).

4. Extended Side Angle (*page 86*).

5. Warrior 1 (*page 52*).

6. Warrior 3 (*page 53*).

7. Seated Spinal Twist (*page 83*).

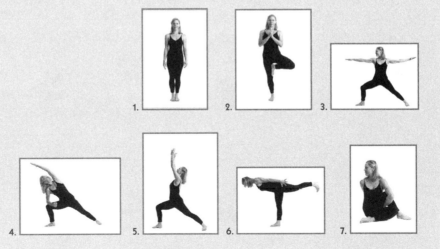

8. Cow Face Pose in a seated pose (*page 84*).

9. Star Pose (*page 60*).

10. Pigeon Pose (*page 62*).

11. Seated Forward Bend (*page 60*).

12. Open Angle Pose (*page 63*).

13. Headstand (*page 73*). Chant *om* in Headstand.

14. Child's Pose (*page 58*).

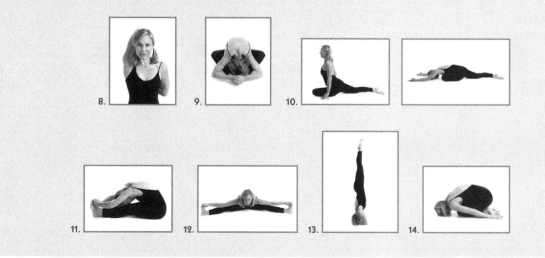

8. 9. 10. 11. 12. 13. 14.

15. Locust Pose (*page 79*).

16. Lion Face (*page 37*).

17. Bow Pose (*page 80*).

18. Bridge Pose (*page 80*).

19. Supine Twist (*page 84*).

20. Come back to seated position.

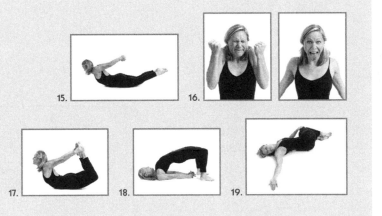

15.

16.

17.

18.

19.

Facial Exercises

1. Temple Dancer Eyes (*page 32*).

2. Puppet Face (*page 19*).

3. Brow Lift (*page 36*).

4. Brushing It Off (*page 96*) Face massage: wipe away the stress from your cheeks and forehead.

5. Ear Pull: the Ear Pull is a form of Indian facial massage/stretching that helps release tension from the jaw and stretches the cartilage under the skin in the surrounding area. It also brings circulation to the face. Simply grab the outer ear rim with the thumb and index of the hand on the same side as the ear you are pulling, and use even strokes from the top of the ear all the way down to the fleshy part of the lobe, pulling outward in rapid, firm movements. This amounts to six or seven pulls on each ear, working from the top to the bottom.

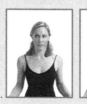 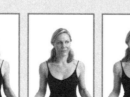 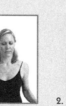 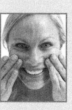 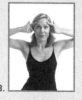

1. 2. 3.

Chakra Meditation

Visualize your first chakra, the Root Chakra, located at the base of the spine. Mentally picture light filling the root center at the base of your spine and pulsating with power. Sit in the center of the heat generated at the base of your spine, and let the energy travel up your spine to the crown of your head.

From a seated position, place your right hand in a fist under your lower ribs as you hollow your belly. Fold forward, head toward the floor, keeping the fist in place.

Corpse Pose (*page 65*).

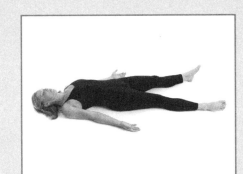

Fire Sequence

The fire sequence is designed to empower and invigorate. It works with heat to charge you up. It will burn off impurities and detoxify. It will clear stagnation and recharge your metabolism. It is appropriate for the morning or the early evening before going out. If you need an energy burst—the yogic equivalent of an espresso—try this one out. It's great to do before going out for a night of dancing, or perhaps a job interview, or anytime you want to transmit self-confidence. Do not practice this sequence before going to bed or if you suffer from insomnia. If the weather is very hot, practice this sequence with caution, but it is a great sequence for when you need to create heat, especially in the winter.

Breathing Practice
Kapalabhati Breathing (*page 108*) five minutes.

Yoga Poses

1. Headstand or modified Headstand (*page 73*), two minutes.

2. Handstand, if desired and accessible (*page 68*).

3. Child's Pose (*page 58*) deep breaths.

4. Warrior 2 (*page 51*) eight counts.

5. Warrior 1 (*page 52*) eight counts.

6. Extended Side Angle Pose (*page 86*) eight counts.

7. Crescent Moon Pose (*page 64*) eight counts.

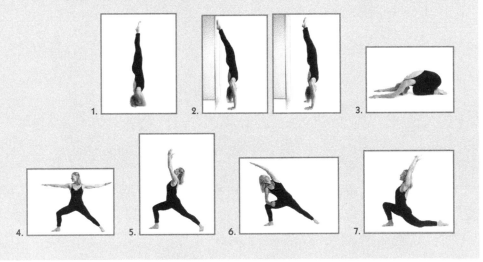

8. Crow Pose (*page 55*) hold as long as you can.

9. Squat with your feet four inches wider than hip-width and place your palms in the center of your chest in prayer position. Place a block under your sit bones or roll a blanket under your heels if you are unable to balance in the squatting position. Practice Kapalabhati Breathing (sixty pumps) then lift your hips, go into a forward bend, and exhale *aaaaah*. Roll up to stand.

10. Now lie facedown on the floor and do the following exercises.

11. Locust Pose (*page 79*) five to eight breaths.

12. Bow Pose (*page 80*) five breaths.

13. Camel Pose (*page 81*) five breaths.

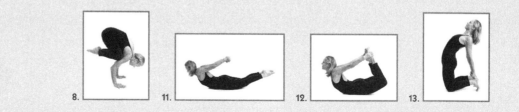

8.   11.   12.   13.

14. Supine Twists (*page 84*) eight breaths.

15. One long, deep Seated Forward Bend (*page 60*) eight breaths.

16. Laughing Yoga: inhale, throw up your arms, and as you exhale, soundlessly laugh. Repeat, then do it again, this time laughing out loud.

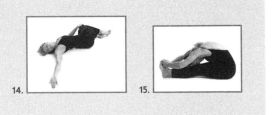

14.

15.

Meditation

Heartbeat Meditation, five minutes.

Sit in a comfortable position. Close your eyes and concentrate on the point between your eyebrows. As you take your inner focus to this spot, begin to breathe in through the nose to a count of four, retain your breath for a count of four, then release your breath to a count of four. Hold out your breath, empty, for four counts. Continue for a total of sixteen rounds.

Now time your four counts with your heartbeat: breathe in for four heartbeats, retain your breath for four heartbeats, then exhale for four heartbeats. Hold out your breath, empty, for four heartbeats. Continue for a total of sixteen rounds, keeping your inner point of concentration at the point between the brows.

Chant

Chant *ram* in Sukhasana, Easy Pose. Five minutes.

Facial Exercises

1. Rub your palms vigorously together and cup them over your eyes for thirty seconds.

2. Satchmo (*page 16*).

3. Baby Bird (*page 27*) three times.

4. Surprise Me! (*page 33*) once.

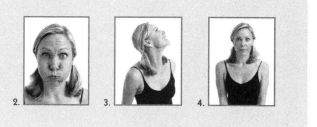

2.   3.   4.

Massage

Foot and Leg Massage

Sit on the floor with your feet together, knees bent, and legs apart, in the shape of a star—Tarasana. You may wish to elevate your seat slightly by placing a rolled-up blanket, bolster, or cushion under the sit bones. Begin by separating your feet slightly and rubbing the balls of both feet with your thumbs and index fingers. Extend the left leg as you keep your right knee bent (Janu Sirsasana legs). Massage your right foot, starting with the inner arch; then work into the middle of the foot in firm, broad strokes. You can dig deeply into the middle of your arch with your index and/or thumb knuckle, and dig another quarter inch to half inch into the center of the foot. This is a strong release point for many, and is associated with the digestive system. "Claw" your heel with your fingernails, digging lightly into the thicker, more callused skin. It will feel good, as the tough skin here can withstand the sensation. Now, turn your foot over and rub the top. Make circular motions at the round joints under each toe, working inside out, from biggest toe to smallest. Rub the indented fleshy space between the joints and ligaments connecting toe to foot at the ankle. Rub the top of the foot gently with thumbs and index fingers.

Continue the massage up the right leg, starting at the back of the ankles, proceeding to the calves (in the belly of the calf muscle) and then down the front of the shin on either side of the shinbone with circular fingertip motions. Apply the knuckles of a lightly fisted right or left hand to the more densely muscular areas, not the bony ones.

Switch your leg position, so that the left leg is extended, and the right knee bent, and apply the same massage techniques to the left foot and calf. Then shake out your legs and extend them. Make fists and gently pummel your legs from the outer bands of the thighs (the IT, or iliotibial, bands) to the outer shins, and work the pummeling motion to the inner calves and then the inner thighs.

This massage sequence can be very brisk, lasting only five minutes, or you can make it luxurious and go for as long as fifteen minutes. You don't need to use massage oil or lotion, especially as dry hands may apply more pressure, but you might want to use either for the legs (oil infused with almond essence is nice for massage; peanut oil is great for stiff joints). If you do use oil, rub it between your hands vigorously to warm it first.

Scalp Massage

In Child's Pose (*see page 58*), rub the thumbs of both hands at the base of the skull, where it attaches to the neck (the occipital ridge), while the index fingers rest on either side of the upper scalp for bracing. Rub the indentations beneath the base of the skull on either side of the upper neck vertebrae, working from the top down to the outer ridges of the vertebrae (you should find a "natural groove"). Pinch the skin between the shoulder blades and the spine with the thumb and index fingers of each hand (the index fingers clasping the upper shoulder, the thumbs pressing the lower), and rub as deeply or gently as feels good. "Shampoo" your scalp with your fingertips, rubbing in circular motions, from the base of the skull to the crown; repeat the motion from the center of the scalp outward until you have covered your entire scalp. Rub your index knuckles in circular motions on your temples lightly, or simply use your fingertips if the knuckle pressure is too intense. Rub the index knuckles into the jaw ridge, starting on the upper jawline beneath the earlobes and running down to the middle point of the chin. Spend a little extra time rubbing the hinge that connects the upper jaw to the lower, using the knuckles of the index fingers for deeper pressure. This massage will take from three to six minutes.

More Meditation

Solar Sunburst

Imagine the light of the sun running from the base of your spine all the way up to your crown, where it beams strong and bright. Suffuse each of your chakras along the way with light. Mentally place yourself within the sunburst. Consider the infinite creativity and energy that burns from your center.

Affirmation

I glow with energy, I shine brightly. (Repeat one to ten times.)

Chant

From Sukhasana, chant *ram* for three to five minutes.

Rest in Corpse Pose (page 65), five to fifteen minutes.

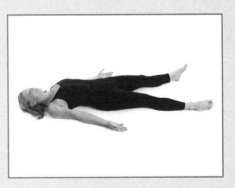

As you may have noticed, each sequence ends with Savasana, Corpse Pose. Savasana is a secret weapon for de-aging, helping slow all the body's functions and facilitating receptivity and release.

chapter nine

Feeding Your Face

These days many of us are confused about how to eat, when to eat, and how much to eat. There seems to be a new diet or eating plan on the market every day. Many of these new plans directly contradict what was in fashion a month or two earlier. An alien scanning the health and nutrition section of any bookstore might deduce that, as a society, we are collectively looking for a quick fix, or some authority to tell us what to do, once and for all. New discoveries prompt a new idea for a miracle diet and a reinvention of the nutritional wheel. Oversimplified "miracle" diets become the diet du jour, attracting die-hard converts, as though eating all green vegetables or only liquefied Brazil nuts were the answer to not only every physical ailment but to all the world's problems. People begin to think the desire for a square meal is a moral weakness!

Added to this is the pressure to meet the demands of a busy daily life. Many of us rush from family duties to work with little time in between. We are grateful for any help that we can get in preparing food. Modern life offers much in the way of convenience—tasty, inexpensive fast food is readily available to most people—but convenience comes with its own set of challenges and pitfalls. Processed fast food is often stripped of nutrients, creating a nutritional imbalance that leads to health-related illnesses such as diabetes, obesity, high cholesterol, and heart disease. And processed foods devoid of the full range of nutrients can play havoc with the skin as well.

Poor nutrition shows up as premature aging on the skin, affecting skin tone, color, and texture. In fact, one of the best ways to anti-age the skin is through eating nourishing and balanced meals.

Because skin is one of the main organs of excretion, poor nutrition leaves its mark on the face right away. Frequent breakouts are often a result of eating sugar and overly processed foods. Sugar is also responsible for rapidly breaking down the cellular structure of the skin, leading to accelerated signs of aging on the face and rest of the body. Dehydration also ages the face dramatically. Drinking excessive caffeine or alcohol or eating excess salt and toxins that lead to dehydration will cause circles and bags under the eyes immediately. When I used to drink a lot of coffee, I started looking like a raccoon in reverse, so dark were the circles under my eyes. Vanity got me to cut down, but I still enjoy a daily cup (it has antioxidants!).

Eating is something we must do to survive, but luckily it's also one of life's greatest pleasures. When done mindfully and with gratitude, it can be a deeply satisfying, absorbing festival for all the senses. Eating can be a sacrament, a celebration, and a moment of peak consciousness and reverence rather than a scattered, hurried act that takes place between mouse clicks and remote-button pushing. Or worse yet, behind the wheel of a car! In fact, if we can simply slow down a bit and think carefully before eating, we can make a huge difference in our health and appearance.

Basic nutrition is not difficult to understand once you have the basics down. We can all eat healthful, balanced meals that nurture both the spirit and the body. And we can all reap the rewards of health and beauty that eating healthfully and mindfully afford. Here are some tips to aid in the process.

Eliminate Distractions

Think of eating a meal as a meditation. Many people don't treat themselves to a pleasurable dining experience because they often eat alone. But eating alone can be a wonderful opportunity for self-nurturing.

Try this as an exercise: think of a meal that you consider truly nurturing and wholesome, and delicious and varied as well. Write out the menu. Shop for the ingredients. Then prepare your food attentively. Enjoy the sensory experience of washing and chopping vegetables and the smells and colors of the food you're preparing. Set the table in an attractive manner. When you sit down to eat, inhale the aroma and appreciate the visual display. Try saying a prayer of thanks for what you are about to eat, and how it will nourish your body and spirit. Thank the earth for providing you with your meal.

Eat with your full attention, in silence, alone. Eat as slowly as you can. Notice the colors, flavors, textures, and aromas. Try chewing each bite of food thirty times. As you chew more slowly, you probably will taste the food more deeply. I tried this exercise the other day as I was eating wild rice and was amazed at how truly nutty it tasted—much more earthy and musky than when I eat quickly. I savored the food and didn't need to eat as much as I would have had I been chewing mindlessly.

Note: *the object of this exercise is to eliminate distractions and concentrate solely on the act of eating, without conversation. It is a Zen-style eating practice, to encourage mindfulness, which is why it is suggested that you do this alone. After you have practiced this once or twice—or maybe even more—feel free to carry this awareness into other daily tasks, and to try carrying aspects of it even when in the presence of others.*

Eliminate Guilt

You deserve to eat well. By nourishing your body and spirit with well-prepared, healthy food, you are honoring yourself. You are creating a healthy body and paving the way for a longer, richer life. This in turn will positively affect those around you, for being healthy, strong, and happy means you can be more present for those you love.

You can eat well and be satisfied. In fact, your life depends upon it. If you are like me, it may take a while to really trust that your body knows what it needs. But if you repress your hunger or try to restrict yourself from what you need, you may toy with your metabolism and experience an energetic backlash. For instance, drinking caffeinated beverages as a meal substitute or appetite suppressant can backfire, as caffeine can affect blood sugar negatively and cause energy crashes. And, as I have mentioned, caffeine's function as a diuretic results in the unfortunate by-product of dehydration.

It's all about balance. Skin, like the rest of our bodies, benefits from a balanced diet comprising a wide range of nutritious foods. And for energy balancing, I find it very helpful to practice yoga or meditate first thing in the morning before eating. You don't have to spend much time on a pre-eating ritual—five to ten minutes of stretching or silent attention to your breath can really help prepare the body for a nice meal.

Then, when you sit down to eat, you'll be more in tune with what your body really needs, and you'll be able to make more conscious choices.

Go for What Calls You

Think of your meal as a sensorial process that starts long before you pick up the fork and take that first bite. The local outdoor farmers' markets are perfect for this kind of eating: browse through the stalls and choose what looks, smells, and feels good to you to eat. What appeals to you visually may very well be what you need nutritionally. Enjoy each of your senses!

If You're Not Hungry, Don't Eat

Sounds simple, right? And yet how many times have you mindlessly noshed, maybe because it was there, or maybe because you were bored or procrastinating on something you needed to do but were avoiding? Also, when the body is tired or dehydrated, it can send out hunger signals (especially sugar cravings) in an attempt to compensate. If you are craving sugar at the end of the day, try to ride it out: drink a glass of water or go to sleep as soon as possible instead. That's what your body really wants. Meditation is another great technique for countering the urge to eat mindlessly. Give yourself five to fifteen minutes to meditate and your craving probably will disappear. Or go for a walk instead. Mindfulness is the key.

It Feels Good to Be Empty

Not for long protracted periods, but enough so that you can tell when you are hungry. You will function more efficiently and have more energy, and your metabolism will work better if you give yourself periods between meals that are long enough to make you really feel ready to eat again.

Whole Food Is Better

The higher your food is in fiber, the longer it takes to digest and be assimilated into the bloodstream. This is good news for your blood sugar: to put it very simply, eating whole foods, such as brown rice instead of white, will make you feel fuller faster, so you'll be less likely to overeat, which will slow down the production of glucose, which in turn will be less likely to convert to fat and skin problems.

The copious quantities of refined sugar in the American diet are responsible for a host of health issues, among them the rise of diabetes. Sugar increases insulin, which may affect the hormones, leading to acne, and also increases inflammation. I have found that when I eat refined sugars, I develop a craving for more of the same and can have trouble curbing the cravings. My skin improved in color and texture when I quit eating refined sugar. Remember, skin is an excretory organ, and the body will shed or sweat out what it can't digest from the pores. That is also why skin can become very oily: any unnecessary fats that the body can't process will end up on the face.

In general, choosing vitamin-packed, nutritive foods with whole grains, minerals, and nutrients will keep blood sugar at a more even keel and reduce weight and bloating all over the face and body. The following are some basic categories of foods that nourish the skin.

Antioxidants

Antioxidants protect the skin from free radicals, which in turn prevents oxidative damage from environmental toxins, the sun, and unhealthy dietary choices. Antioxidants can help assist in the prevention of disease, especially cancer.

Antioxidants, which include vitamins A, C, and E and selenium, are found in a variety of foods:

Vitamin A in sweet potatoes, carrots, butternut squash
Vitamin C in citrus fruits, tomatoes, and berries
Vitamin E in wheat germ, almonds, and peaches
Selenium in turkey, tuna, and cottage cheese

Omega-3 Fatty Acids

Omega-3 fatty acids help protect the skin and are healthful for the entire body. These acids are found in salmon, walnuts, flaxseeds and oil, and omega-3–fortified eggs. Because they produce a sense of satiety, omega-3 fatty acids are an integral part of a well-rounded, nourishing diet. Furthermore, they may help prevent cravings for unhealthy foods.

Dark Greens

Dark leafy greens and cruciferous vegetables are wonderful for the regeneration of the cells. The oxygenating properties of these foods help to kick-start the mitochondria, the powerhouses of the cells. So eating kale, spinach, lettuce, and broccoli will help to keep your skin cells regenerating. Freshly juiced, these greens are delicious (especially with a squeeze of lemon and ginger for detoxification), and you will see the effects right away as your skin brightens and clears.

Dairy

Dairy is excellent for the skin. Dairy contains high levels of skin-nourishing zinc (which can also be found in grains and cruciferous vegetables). You can derive great benefit from eating yogurt, which, because of its healthy bacteria and culture, is thought to be highly nourishing for the skin cells. In Ayurvedic treatment—based on traditional Indian medicine—the fat that dairy contains is considered a building block for the tissues, and therefore it helps to restore the skin. Many European traditional skin-care treatments revolve around milk.

Liquids and Foods High in Water

Lettuce, melons, and cucumbers are all cooling foods high in water that act as diuretics. They will relieve bloating and flush toxins and create a sense of fullness when eaten. They hydrate the skin marvelously. Hydrated skin is an excellent foil to facial aging, as it prevents dryness, and it also helps the skin to receive nutrients from food.

The best way to hydrate your skin is to drink plenty of water. Drink as much water as you reasonably can. It is preferable to drink water at room temperature, as this is compatible with your body's internal temperature so it won't shock your internal organs with a radical temperature change. However, iced beverages are delicious and refreshing on hot days.

Drink filtered water whenever possible. This will help to eliminate environmental toxins from what you drink and, by extension, filter what your organs and skin absorb. Buy water filters and filter your water at home. You can carry your filtered water with you in a portable, reusable bottle. This is better for your body and the environment than buying bottled water, which is often not as clean as the manufacturers would have you think.

Drinking herbal teas is a great way to get valuable hydration and delicious taste. They quench the thirst and can satisfy the palate. Since the body craves sweets when it's dehydrated, if you are craving a sweet treat, an herbal tea can do the trick. Cinnamon is a great natural sweetener and is also delicious as an iced or hot tea. You may purchase any herbal teas containing cinnamon that are on the market (I like Bengal Spice by Celestial Seasonings, or Yogi Tea)—or, if you choose, brew your own by bringing about six to eight cups of water to a boil over the stove, then adding three or four cinnamon sticks, and letting it steep on a low heat, uncovered, for about twenty minutes. You may also add other spices (about a teaspoon or so) of any or all of the following: cloves, ginger, nutmeg, and cardamom. Then turn off the heat and let the tea sit for a minute or two. Pour your tea through a strainer and enjoy. You may also pour some warm milk into the tea for more of a traditional Indian chai. This tea is also good iced. On a hot summer day, peppermint tea is especially delicious iced.

Anyone can grow a few fresh herbs in their kitchen: mint is especially easy to grow, and can be used in many dishes as a cooling, refreshing note and is delicious when paired with creamy foods such as yogurt.

Lemon verbena is a delicately scented herb that is delicious in teas as well. Or try growing some purple basil and adding fresh leaves to a tomato salad or a Thai stir fry. Lavender can be a piquant counterpoint to sweet custards and is also good in small amounts in fruit salads.

Think of eating well as preventative medicine: when you nourish your body with the nutrients it needs and craves, you will create balance in your body and in your life. As you become more attuned to what your body needs and loves to eat, you will intuitively move away from unhealthy eating. If you occasionally backslide, your skin will react because you'll be less tolerant of toxins. As you get cleaner, your body will become averse to what it used to not mind. Think of your health as constantly evolving: it is a work in progress that continues to be refined with practice.

The more balance and awareness you bring into eating, the more positive benefits the skin will enjoy. Remember that what you feed your body will also feed your face, so nourish your skin with a wide variety of healthful, fresh, and delicious meals.

chapter ten

Icing the Cake: Natural Beauty Products and Supplements

In Chapter Nine, we looked at how what we choose to feed our bodies is directly reflected in our faces. Now let's turn to what we put *on* our faces. Your skin "eats" nutrients through the pores. What you place upon your skin's surface absorbs into your bloodstream (think of topical pain medications) and then in turn will feed your internal organs, muscles, nerves, and connective tissue. This is why choosing skin products that are made of organic ingredients is so much healthier for your skin. Organic ingredients contain up to twenty-five percent more antioxidants, for example. And do you really want your skin to ingest the unpronounceable chemicals that are listed on the sides of the bottles of so many "beauty treatments" we see today?

Luckily, more and more companies are producing very high quality pure skin treatment lines in recognition of what is becoming abundantly clear: if it's not something you would eat through your mouth, you shouldn't make your pores, skin, and internal organs eat it either.

The six topical steps (and corresponding types of products) for maintaining and improving the skin are cleansing, sloughing, purifying, refining, moisturizing, and protecting.

Cleansing

Cleansing is the first (and arguably most important) step, as it primes the canvas of the skin. Cleansing removes bacteria, excess oils, and dirt. It actually can be a damaging process if the wrong products are used. Many over-the-counter products are too potent, laden with chemicals that strip the skin of its natural protective coat (the sebum) and dry it unnecessarily. Look for a mild, gentle cleanser that doesn't contain harsh chemical ingredients (one with fruit acids is great for sloughing off accumulated dead skin cells). There are some excellent vegetable-based soaps (especially olive oil) that are wonderful for the skin. I like a face wash that contains fruit acids; for my skin type (which is a combination of oily and normal) this is excellent, as it mildly sloughs off dead skin.

To cleanse, rub your fingertips in a circular, light motion on the surface of moist skin (avoid overly hot water—warm water is best), including the neck and throat areas. Apply upward sweeps rather than downward strokes. To shrink the pores, splash cold water on your face when you rinse. When you are finished cleansing, lightly pat the skin dry with a clean towel. Patting the skin lets your circulation rise toward the surface of your skin, bringing a rosy glow and more oxygen.

Face washing is one of the main ways we touch our faces—usually at least twice a day. For this reason, cleansing is a great opportunity to use mindful, loving touch on your beautiful face. Because it's something you do all the time, you can observe your normal method and start to make improvements right away. By refining your cleansing method, you will definitely see changes in the appearance of your facial skin.

If you cleanse deeply and thoroughly before bed and you frequently change your linens, you don't have to wash your face again first thing in the morning. You haven't gotten dirty sleeping, and there is no need to strip the skin of its protective mantle. Wait until your skin has sweat to wash your face again—maybe after a workout.

When cleansing the skin of your body, the same principles apply. Do not be overly aggressive in scrubbing your skin. Take the opportunity to celebrate yourself in your bathing rituals. The ancient yogis considered cleanliness, or *saucha*, an important observance (*niyama*) on the path of yoga. Bathing is still considered sacred in India, and rubbing the body with oil before a bath is considered auspicious. While bathing, prayers are said to bless the cleansing ritual. Baths are considered much more cleansing than showers, and constitute a large portion of Ayurvedic (Indian medicine) practice. We can all benefit from ritualizing our cleansing time, using it to make ourselves sweeter on the inside as well as the outside. When scrubbing your body (perhaps with a loofah or washcloth), try singing or chanting. Rub your body gently, and then take a bath. You may add essential oils, milk, or a handful of fresh herbs to the bath. You can also draw the bath, then after the water has stopped running, add an herbal tea bag (chamomile, mint, or an herbal fruit tea such as apricot, strawberry, or raspberry) and let yourself steep in the concoction. Two or three drops of essential oils such as lemon, orange, mint, lavender, juniper, or basil are also an excellent addition to a hot bath.

To further ritualize your bath and make it into a mini-retreat, try turning off the lights and bathing by candlelight, and continue singing, chanting, or playing inspirational music. When you are washing your hair, rinse your head in the coldest water you can stand to add shine and luster. After your bath, rub your body with a sweet natural oil as well. While massaging your skin, pay attention to any sore spots. Give the places that are sensitive tender loving care in the form of your touch.

Preparing treatments at home can be a fun and spiritual way to connect with the sacred goddess of beauty.

Believe it or not, it is actually pretty simple to make many skin treatments at home. (If you are pressed for time, or just not a kitchen person, you can purchase fresh, natural, organic products in small enough amounts that they will not expire.)

You can try making your own Ayurvedic soap from a mix of one cup of pure, unscented, natural liquid soap, adding one-half cup of water or herbal tea, and five drops of essential oil. You may use a combination of oils, but do not exceed five drops of essential oil total. Oils that work well include ylang-ylang (good for calming nerves, high blood pressure), wintergreen (heals skin ailments), sandalwood (used to help sensitive skin and to heal stretch marks), grapefruit (helpful for sore and stiff muscles, acne), dark patchouli (acne, nerves), lavender (calming), peppermint (adds heat), tea tree (for acne and oily skin), eucalyptus (burns, insect bites), chamomile (anti-inflammatory), geranium (calming), and rose (nourishing for skin).

One last point: your sinuses can also use a cleansing! The yogis devised the neti pot for those who suffer from congestion and sinus problems. Make a mixture of pure, warm filtered water and a pinch of sea salt, tip your head back, and gently pour some water from the neti pot through one nostril, then expel it through the other. Repeat on the other side. You will feel relief instantly and experience a reduction of the swelling of the nose's mucus membranes. Using a neti pot will also reduce inflammation and clear up your breathing if you are congested. The action of inhaling and exhaling water mixed with pure sea salt will also tone the flesh around your nose, making it firmer and less prone to drooping.

Sloughing

Removing accumulated dead cells from the top layer of skin is important to do on a regular basis. Various spots and discolorations can be removed with conscientious yet gentle sloughing. Fruit is a great ingredient to look for in any sloughing product. The acids in fruit are helpful for removing dull, discolored outer layers that are trapped on the surface of the skin, and will reveal a fresher, more youthful new layer.

All fruits produce acids, but pineapple, papaya, strawberry, apricot, and blueberry are particularly good for the skin. There are many fantastic face scrubs on the market, and you certainly can make your own scrubs as well. Using scrubs is a great way to exfoliate the skin, again helping remove old, trapped skin cells and reveal more youthful, glowing skin. Be mindful when using a scrub to not scrub too vigorously, and always avoid the delicate skin beneath the eyes.

Ground oats and almonds in equal ratio moistened with a little water make a good scrub. Use whole oats, not instant! Ground walnut shells have traditionally been used in scrubs, as they are both sloughing and moisturizing and are good exfoliators, but used too frequently or with too much pressure they can be harsh and drying. A popular scrub that can be found in several different lines is one made of apricot and walnut shells. Go easy here if you have dry or sensitive skin.

You may also make a scrub from flour and water (or, if your skin is dry, milk) and scrub the paste on the skin with a loofah or sea sponge before bathing. If you are thin and tend toward dryness, try a paste made with chickpea, millet, or oat flour, almond, sesame or coconut oil, and milk. If you are medium build and energetic, try barley or rice flour with milk. If you tend to be slower and more mellow, your constitution will benefit from corn or millet flour mixed with clay and water.

Salt scrubs really slough the body of its dead skin and moisturize at the same time, leaving the skin soft and dewy like a baby's. There are many wonderful products on the market now, or you can go to a spa and have a body scrub treatment. Sugar is commonly used in body scrubs, as it is a powerful ingredient for removing trapped debris on the epidermis. I use a homemade solution of sea salt, mint, and oil and lightly massage and scrub my entire body with it after a good soak in the bath, when the skin has softened up. I will put a little scrub on the soles of my feet and lightly pumice. If you prefer to go deeper to draw up impurities from under the pores, use a mask. Masks cleanse deeply and draw out what is beneath the topmost layer of the skin. They can also be deeply hydrating, as they may be left on the skin for longer periods and hydrate or nourish through the pores to the cells beneath the epidermis. You can make a mask for yourself with any of several fruits—strawberry, banana, pineapple, or papaya. Simply mash up enough fruit to constitute a small serving and spread it all over your freshly cleaned face. You may wish to add a little bit of ground oats as a binder, and also to allow for exfoliation when you remove the mask. Let the mask sit for about five minutes, then add a little water and gently scrub the concoction in spiral motions with your fingers as you rinse. Papaya is my favorite fruit for a mask, as it has very strong enzymes that will break down dead, dull skin beautifully.

Purifying

Clay is a classic deep cleanser that leaches impurities out from under the skin's surface and dries off excess oils that can trap dirt. For those with large pores that clog easily, a good clay mask will immeasurably improve the texture and appearance of the skin. The pores will shrink and refine. Choose a green or red clay product; or make one of your own by purchasing dry clay at a health food store—just add enough water to make a smooth paste, and apply. If you live in an area where you can find clay, you can forage some and use it on your skin. In Big Sur, California, you can find wonderful clay, the same kind that Native Americans used in their rituals. Obviously, you will want to go for the purest local natural clay you can find—the farther from the reach of human hands, the better.

Steaming is also a great way to open the pores and sweat out impurities. Be careful that you don't steam for too long (no more than fifteen minutes maximum), as you will dry out your skin after a certain point. Be sure to drink a lot of water after. You can steam your entire face and body in a spa setting (spraying water mixed with a little eucalyptus will work as an antiseptic) or you can steam your face, throat, and neck at home. Boil a large pot of water, then pour it into a large bowl. Choose two teaspoons of fresh herbs or two drops of essential oil that target your particular skin concern (for detoxifying, rosemary is particularly good) and add it to the water. You can also use a mint tea bag if you don't have fresh herbs. Place a towel over your head, lean over the bowl, and let your skin drink in the warm, aromatic vapors. Don't get too close, or you will feel your skin "burn" (about six inches from the water is safe). After you have steamed for five to fifteen minutes, splash the skin with cool water and apply a toner. Finish with a light moisturizer.

Refining

Toners work to refine the skin and close the pores after a deep cleansing. They remove excess oil and brighten the skin. Toners can be used after deep cleansing and/or throughout the day. In the afternoon, it is preferable to tone the skin rather than subject it to a full wash with a cleanser, as this will not strip the skin unnecessarily.

If your skin is oily or combination, use some toner in between cleansing and moisturizing. You may use a mildly astringent toner that helps to brace the skin—chamomile, lavender, and calendula are all good natural components. Choose an organic toner from your local health food store that contains ingredients suitable for your particular skin type. Diluted tea tree oil is an excellent antibacterial and is good for people who are prone to acne and breakouts. If you have normal or dry skin, you can also benefit from using a toner, but make sure you choose one that has less astringent properties, such as a rose-water-based solution. You can also use a bit of toner throughout the day to refresh your skin and take off accumulated dirt, debris, and perspiration. After a brief toner break, make sure to reapply some sunscreen with an SPF of 15 (if you have oily skin, don't go higher, the SPFs over 15 tend to be too thick and will clog your pores).

Moisturizing

Your skin should be a little damp when you apply your moisturizer. Most people use too much product, which can result in a greasy face that hasn't really absorbed anything. Be sparing and remember, less is more. Sweep the surface of your skin with light, upward strokes of the index and middle fingers. Think of this as a type of light massage, and let your circulation rise to the surface of the skin. Then tap your skin with your index and middle fingers to help the pores absorb the moisturizer or oil. Your pores will "drink" the treatment better if you tap, and this will help you to avoid wasting the product on the surface of the skin. If your skin looks very shiny after applying your moisturizer, it hasn't absorbed all the product. Tap the skin until the bulk of the shininess is gone. You may finish with light pats on the surface of the skin, again to bring up circulation and rosiness to the face.

Olive oil and other pure, high-quality carrier oils (apricot, almond, coconut) are some of nature's best moisturizers. Quality is the key in purchasing oil for the skin. Make sure your oil is organic and cold pressed if possible, and check to make sure it hasn't been exposed to a lot of light (a dark bottle kept in a cool place is preferable). Apricot, almond, and coconut oils are all excellent for the skin, and can be applied sparingly to the surface of the face after cleansing. Scenting oils with the essence of plants or flowers can tweak the oil for a customized purpose. Here is a list of herbs and flowers that you can add (in oil form) to a base oil for specific results:

Calendula: anti-inflammatory
Lavender: soothing, mildly antiseptic
Tea tree oil: strong antibacterial; very good for oily skin—use in small amounts
Rosemary: cleansing
Rose: nourishing
Orange: antidepressant, toning

Lemon: energizing, astringent

Neroli: a miracle oil for reducing puffiness; also smells delicious and is calming and sensual

Shea butter is another fantastic natural moisturizer. It is very rich, and can be used as a moisturizer for the hair, skin, lips, and, in small amounts, on the face. Shea oil can go bad quickly, so make sure it is kept cool and out of the light.

Honey is one of nature's miracle foods for the body and the skin. You can make a mask of yogurt and honey to moisturize and protect the skin. Mix one-quarter cup of yogurt with two rounded tablespoons of raw honey. Apply to the skin of the face, throat, and neck, and let sit for five to ten minutes. Propolis is produced by bees and works to seal the skin from unwanted elements. You can also eat propolis to boost your immune system and get a nice energy buzz.

An avocado mask is great for making the skin buttery and baby soft. Just mash up half of a ripe avocado and apply it to your face. Leave it on for about ten minutes, then wash it off, pat your face dry, and moisturize lightly.

Protecting

No section on skin care and beauty would be complete without a mention of protection for the skin. Protecting your skin from the sun's damaging rays is the single most important way to prevent aging on the surface of the skin.

Unfortunately, we are living in an era of increased UV exposure. Not only is this a potential threat to our lives (in the form of skin cancer), but overexposure to UV light from the sun's rays causes the worst (and most easily avoided) form of premature aging, and the most telling one, too. Get in the habit of applying an SPF-enriched moisturizer (15 is the best), not just on your face, but on your hands, arms, and anywhere else that receives the sun's attention. You can also wear a hat with a brim, gloves, and light long sleeves in the heat. Consider carrying an attractive parasol on warm, sunny days, and wear sunglasses that screen ultraviolet rays to avoid developing crow's-feet. Recently Madonna was photographed on the beach in a caftan that resembled a Bedouin tribal garment. While this may be rather extreme, she has certainly defied popular notions of what attractive at almost fifty can be.

Face and Body Food

The skin absorbs and ingests nutrients through the pores. You can feed your skin the same way you feed your stomach. There are many natural ingredients and foods that the skin absorbs easily—this is one of the reasons that Ayurvedic medicine employs fortified oils as a treatment.

In choosing ingredients for your face, here are some general guidelines:

Rosemary: tones, purifies

Yogurt: moisturizes, softens

Coconut: softens

Peppermint: tones

Lemon: tones, alleviates depression

Lavender: detoxifies, energizes

Verbena: tones

Pineapple, papaya, strawberry, and blueberry contain fruit acids and antioxidants that slough dead skin cells. Mash up enough fruit for a small serving and spread it all over your face as a mask after cleansing. Let sit for five to ten minutes, then rinse. Pat skin, then apply a light moisturizer of your choice.

Cucumber reduces bloating. The old classic of placing slices over the eyes will alleviate bags, but you can spread pureed cucumber over your entire face for the same effect. Eating cucumber will help reduce general bloating and puffiness.

Oatmeal, almond, apricot, and finely crushed walnut shells are all good scrub ingredients to slough and polish the skin.

Carrot and pumpkin both have a lovely, buttery quality when pureed and applied to the skin. The vitamin A that these foods contain is especially nourishing and helps the skin soften and break down dead skin. Place two or three carrots and a teaspoon of tahini in a food processor and puree. If using pumpkin, use fresh pumpkin (about a quarter of a cup) and puree in a food processor. Try a puree of carrot and tahini as a softening, mask, or look for moisturizers that contain these delicious natural foods for the skin. Use these moisturizers on the soles of the feet and the hands.

Persimmon has intensely hydrating properties, and when combined with rose geranium, it is a great anti-inflammatory. You can look for a moisturizer containing these at your local health food store.

Moisturizing sprays made of purified water or water mixed with a little rose or orange blossom water, mint, or citrus essence are great used at any point in the day. Burt's Bees and Evian also make some good ones. Your skin needs a drink on a hot day, just like your body!

Acupuncture

After cleansing and moisturizing, you are ready to do some acupressure, massage, and/ or several facial exercises. You may also consider going to see an acupuncturist to deepen your facial rejuvenation. Acupuncture for the face has long been employed in the East, but Westerners are now starting to discover its power. You can go to an experienced acupuncturist and have a "facelift" through the skillful application of tiny needles on the surface of your face. In addition to stimulating major nodes of energy and healing, this type of treatment gives the face a more youthful lift that will last several weeks.

Makeup

Playing with your facial appearance through the artful use of makeup is a skill we can all refine. No matter how adept you are, it's always possible to learn new tricks. Also, we can become so accustomed to seeing ourselves in a certain way that we no longer really see ourselves objectively.

Or perhaps your self-image is frozen in a time and place no longer reflective of reality (many people seem to get trapped in a certain era of style, usually the one in which they felt the most vibrant and attractive or the one in which they defined their personal style). One of the biggest tip-offs of age and aging is dressing in the style of an outmoded decade, without a hint of irony. We have all seen this in friends and family members . . . the immobile, omnipresent bouffant (circa 1961) of Aunt Gladys, or perhaps it's Uncle Phil's polyester bell-bottom houndstooth leisure suit in orange and brown (circa 1974). I am not suggesting you be a slave to fashion—far from it. Rather, develop a classic sense of what works for you and be open to trying new things. In the area of makeup, for example, using lip color is an easy and inexpensive way to update your look. As we age, our skin tone begins to dull and flatten as a result of a loss of collagen, so bright, contrasty shades tend to look glaring. Go with subtle tones that are in your skin's natural color range. Olive- and brown-toned complexions can wear soft corals and gold tones. Ivory and pink tones can wear colors in the warm violet and red range. In general, picking your best facial feature and accenting it is a good strategy. Less is more, and a simple accent of the mouth, cheekbones, or eyes can be quite striking.

Invest in a tinted moisturizer with an SPF of 15. If you were to choose one single product, this would be the best makeup you could possibly wear. Rather than applying a foundation, then a moisturizer, then an SPF, combining these three functions in one product will give you an excellent way to cover your bases (pun intended). Choose a tint that matches your skin tone as closely as possible (going in the sun with the product near your jaw is a good way to test it). I really like Benefit's You Rebel, which is light and moist and has a bit of a warmish gold cast to it. It matches my skin well in the warmer months and gives me a natural, sun-kissed glow. As skin ages, it becomes less lustrous and light reflective (again, due to collagen loss), so avoid dry, powdery products on the face. Blotting with a tissue is a good alternative to powdering the skin, which can leave a dreaded crepe-type finish. Avoid blush altogether, as it tends to look garish on aging skin. The excellent skin tone you will develop from the Yoga Face (particularly from the inversions such as Downward-Facing Dog and Headstand) will give you a naturally rosy glow.

If you have deep-set eyes, or if you have begun to develop lines around your eyes, avoid wearing liner around the lower lids, as it will make your eyes look smaller. Line the upper lids' lash lines very judiciously and your eyes will look larger.

Curl your lashes with a high-quality lash curler, then sweep a small amount of mascara from the base of the lash to the outer edge, curling the wand as you go to the end of the lash. Distribute the bulk of the mascara to the outer lash rather than the base, where it will gunk and clump.

Eyebrows are the frames of the face and can create dramatic changes in facial appearance. A high, semicircular arch will give you a youthful quality. Keep your eyebrows well groomed, but do not overpluck, as eyebrow hairs don't always grow back. Overplucked, sparse eyebrows are very aging, and, in fact, a thicker eyebrow makes you look younger. Do not draw your eyebrows on; if you must augment your natural line, use a high-quality eyebrow brush and some eyebrow shadow. Choose a brow shade that complements your natural hair color, and definitely do not do dark brown or black eyebrows with platinum hair (sable looks best on highlighted blondes). Moisten the brush, then extend your natural line to obtain more natural results.

Highlight

I am a huge fan of highlight rather than shadow, as it pops and opens the facial areas you wish to showcase. Eyes, lips, and cheeks are all brilliantly illuminated by the artful application of a little highlight. And unlike blushes, eyeshadows, dark lipsticks, and other darkening forms of makeup, highlights brighten and expose the facial features without closing them in and overly defining them. As we age, our skin loses luster, and the last thing most of us need is to further darken and narrow the features. Highlight always occurs near shadow, so look for the areas above where shadows naturally occur on your face (the brow bone, above the cheekbone, under the orbital bone, down the center of the bridge of the nose, the center of the lips, the center of the chin, on the inner edges of the outer forehead, and above the jaw ridge) when looking for places to add a little subtle shimmer. You can apply a little dab of highlight in the center of the eyelid or under the brow bone to brighten and awaken your facial features. A hint of highlight above the cheekbone can counter a gaunt appearance in the cheeks. Similarly, a bit of highlight down the bridge of the nose can add a bit of contour to the facial appearance (keep this subtle and save it for glamorous nights on the town). Highlight on the center of the lower lip is also a beautiful effect, as it plumps the mouth. A cream highlight applied with a sponge-tipped wand can look dewy and moist, as opposed to a powder, which can be drying.

Supplements

It is best to eat a varied and balanced diet full of unprocessed and organic foods that are rich in fiber. The body absorbs nutrients from food better than from pills and powders, and many supplements are hard to absorb. Pills and tablets can be hard to metabolize, and often their ingredients are eliminated before they are absorbed. However, supplements can be beneficial when used judiciously.

Minerals are necessary to revitalize skin as it ages. As we age, the mitochondria, the powerhouses of the cells, begin to slow their activity. Thus minerals are vital in helping to recharge the cells. Sulfur- and mineral-rich green powerhouse foods such as spirulina and algae work as antioxidants, helping to counter the effects of free radicals and are therefore anti-aging miracle supplements. Make a fresh fruit smoothie with green minerals to reenergize your cells and have a power-charged day. Drinking the juice of green vegetables with some ginger and lemon is an excellent skin cocktail and will also give you a pure, powerful energy boost.

Sulfur is an excellent supplement to take orally to aid in remineralizing the skin. Highly effective sulfur supplements include alpha-lipoic acid, chondroitin, and glucosamine sulfate (also thought to help the joints and to counter inflammation).

Propolis, honey, and ginseng are all powerful energizers and revitalizers when taken as supplememts. Propolis is also a powerful natural sealant when applied topically. Sea algae is fantastic for remineralization of the skin's surface. Look for beauty treatments and topical creams that contain these vital skin nourishers. I like Dr. Alkaitis's organic face treatment line, as it contains high quantities of sea minerals.

Calcium and magnesium are good for maintaining bone density, and when taken in combination are more effective. Take in a liquid form if possible and before bed to aid in sleep. Iron is vital for the production of red blood cells, which on the face can translate as a rosier complexion. Get iron in your diet by eating lots of dark leafy greens and black beans. Cook on a cast-iron skillet.

Moderate vitamin supplementation can be a wise choice for the skin. Vitamin C can boost the immune system and help revitalize the skin. Vitamin A is an antioxidant that can be found in eggs and fish. When present in the diet it can help reverse cancerous changes in the cells. Vitamin E is also an antioxidant that protects lipids (the building blocks of the cell membranes) from oxidation and damage from free radicals (toxins caused by environmental exposure and diet). Current research shows that Vitamin E is better absorbed through nutrition than topically.

Sleep and Rest

Sleep deprivation accelerates the aging process. Puffy eyes, dark circles, and dehydrated skin are all telltale signs that the body hasn't gotten enough rest. The body does most of its repairing during deep sleep (even the spinal cord gets longer at night, as the intervertebral discs plump in slumber), so this is the time to turn back the clock and maximize nocturnal repair.

Signal to your body and mind that it's time to wind down by taking a lavender-scented bath before bed. Then apply a moisturizer that will sink in and repair your skin while you doze. An under-eye-gel will take away puffiness. A hydrating night cream will rejuvenate the face. A deeply moisturizing hand cream applied before bed will impart youth to your appearance (it's said that hands always give away age—not so with nightly moisturizing treatments!). Try a deeply moisturizing foot cream before bed, and enhance the treatment by wearing socks!

A gentle yet effective skin maintenance regimen like the one I have outlined will help to add a new level of luster to your face. In addition, you can artfully apply a little makeup to help highlight the features you wish to accent and to diminish what you'd rather downplay. Sleeping regularly and well will help to set all the good work you've been doing. Using these strategies, your face will accurately reveal how you feel inside: ageless and timeless!

chapter eleven

Inner Beauty/
Outer Beauty

The Yoga Face program encourages glowing, radiant health from the inside out. Beauty is a facet of the brilliant jewel of health: as your health increases, your outer appearance shines more brightly in direct proportion to it. But for many, the idea of beauty seems unattainable. We truly become beautiful once we stop looking for it outside ourselves and turn our searching gaze deep within.

As a young actress, I had the opportunity to learn a lot about how we as a culture relate to the concept of beauty. After completing a prestigious actors' conservatory training program, I was to be photographed for my headshots. It was my first time, and I was anxious and self-conscious, fretting that I wasn't "model perfect." I was interested in developing a stage career and didn't feel comfortable with being scrutinized up close. And I was intimidated by all the beautiful, slick head shots of movie star types, grinning like cats with canary feathers between their teeth, that I saw at the head-shot photographer's studio. I knew I wasn't the supermodel type, so I decided to let my head-shot photo session be an opportunity to act myself into beauty. Instead of sending myself negative messages about how imperfect I was, before the session I nurtured myself, meditated, went running, and ate well.

The photographer flirted with me during the session, which made me feel a bit tense and nervous, until I stumbled upon a huge discovery: if I focused (forgive the pun) on the photographer and my relationship to him, rather than obsessing on how I was being perceived, I could really enjoy what was taking place. By flirting with me, the photographer was trying to give me a sense of confidence and playfulness. When I got out of myself and decided to give back to the photographer, I totally relaxed. I made the choice to positively respond to his cheesy pickup lines (he wasn't really trying to pick me up; he just wanted to get some good shots) and everything transformed.

A week went by, and when I saw the pictures, I was thrilled. The shots that the camera caught me flirting in really were beautiful. I learned that day that cameras (like people) pick up on the energy you transmit. The camera reads mood and thought, much more than proportion and line. It is amazing how people who are technically beautiful (meaning their proportions are what we define as classically perfect) don't always photograph as beautiful, whereas some ordinary people will photograph brilliantly.

There are many examples of this "star quality" in people who are not classically beautiful. Look at a photograph of Eleanor Roosevelt: she dedicated her life to being of service and helping others, and she positively glowed. She was magnetic and beautiful, though nowhere near "pretty." Or look at some of the old, unretouched studio publicity shots of the Hollywood greats: before retouching, Bette Davis was certainly no ravishing beauty, but she truly transmitted glamour in every scene she played.

This is the case with many magnetic and charismatic people: though not stereotypically beautiful, they radiate energy, charisma, and charm. That's why it can be disconcerting to see a celebrity in real life—we are shocked when they don't look like what we imagined. And who among us hasn't secretly delighted when we've seen a god or goddess of beauty brought down to size in an unflattering candid shot, or spied a celebrity demigod on the street in sweats and a baseball cap? More than just schadenfreude at seeing their imperfections, it's a relief on some level to know that those "perfect" beings are human, just like the rest of us.

Beauty is a fluid notion—it responds to our ever-shifting perceptions, as well as to larger cultural forces and trends that sometimes are beyond our personal control. For example, plump bodies have always been fashionable when food is scarce, and certain tones of skin color have gone from being the ideal to the loathed, and back again. Our own self-image can fluctuate as much as the weather—"bad hair days" can wreak havoc on social plans.

That being said, there are real and definite methods for increasing outer beauty. Yes, true beauty emerges from inside, but the face and body encase our inner beauty, and must be maintained and nurtured as well. Most people are put off by a ramshackle exterior when they are house shopping, no matter how much the realtor insists the place has "good bones."

And one thing I've learned as a performer is that people often find self-expression from the outside in. The great acting legend Laurence Olivier was just this type of actor: he was no Stanislavsky-based method actor, finding his way from the inside out. He came from the grand traditions of the British stage, going back hundreds of years to Shakespeare's time. For Olivier, outer physical transformation was how he approached the inner character. In other words, the outer shell *was* the man. In his book on acting, he wrote that for him the key to finding a character was in "finding the nose." When he was playing Richard the Third at the Old Vic, and later on film, he started by sculpting a nose out of modeling putty, and for him this one detail *made* him the into character.

I have had this experience both on stage and in life: what woman doesn't know that finding the right shoes can be truly transformative? (Look at Cinderella!) This shoe adage is an old chestnut in stage circles as well: finding "the walk" is another essential component of building a character. Try it yourself: watch the way people walk when you are out in public. Look at people from behind as they walk down the street. You can probably guess age, social station, income, and how that person feels about himself just by watching his gait. That's why the postural benefits of the physical poses contribute to a more youthful look—they help your posture. Another example is hair: I recently had the privilege of being a hair model for an excellent stylist who gave me beautiful hair extensions. I was shocked at how much more youthful I felt with a full, long head of bright blond hair!

So it's not really superficial to care about the surface, since it provides us and others with a clue as to who we are and what matters to us. No matter what features and attributes we're born with, an accurate assessment of our assets can help us present ourselves in our best light. We can also skillfully downplay the attributes we aren't as happy with. But no matter what, we can all do something about our bodies, skin, hair, and teeth. It can be unsettling to observe a person who is bedraggled, messy, or unkempt, since we know that these basics of self-care represent mental as well as physical well-being. It's all about balance. And not only is taking care of your appearance fun and creative, it can truly be an art.

So many people limit themselves in their look. Many of us hang on to outdated beliefs about what we are, negative comments made in passing by jealous rivals or judgmental authority figures. Or perhaps we got an unflattering picture taken and are convinced that's how we really look all the time. Sometimes I think people hang on to low-self-esteem patterns and negative self-talk because it is easier to be negative and self-pitying than to actually do something. Or perhaps we are invested in staying "unattractive" because the prospect of claiming our physical beauty is somehow frightening.

I can remember receiving a negative message from my mother when I was five years old. I was admiring my pretty braids in the mirror and my mother told me to stop being vain. I asked her what vain meant. I got the impression it wasn't a good thing to be. It wasn't wrong of my mother to try to encourage me to not be superficial; she was trying to show me that physical beauty was not the most important thing of all, and yet I somehow translated this to mean it was bad to be proud of my appearance. I also have been hassled on the street by members of the opposite sex to the point that I would deliberately downplay my appearance to be left alone.

But the truth is, we women pass a lot of judgment on ourselves as well. Most men I talk to tell me they prefer a woman with some shape to a narrow, rail-like stick figure. Yet, often, women will express the tyranny of body judgment on themselves and one another quite mercilessly. The kind of appreciation I have gotten from the opposite sex as I have aged has been more respectful and heartfelt, perhaps because I respect myself more. I am not saying I don't miss the days when I could wear just about anything and carry it off, but I must say I enjoy the flip side, which is feeling totally comfortable without a drop of makeup on and wearing flip flops instead of heels.

Part of building a healthy sense of self-esteem around personal image is to start to approach it as a game or a creative exercise. The following exercise will help you to see how you define yourself, and it will provide you with some clues as to how to expand and update your personal image. Think of this image-shaping portion of the Yoga Face as an acting exercise—you are not tied to your choices for perpetuity, but rather your identity can be a fluid one that metamorphoses as you do. Or, even better, get in touch with that kid who used to love to play dress-up and be different characters. (If you never did that as a kid, now's your chance. It's fun!)

Symbolic Self-Portrait

Try this exercise. Write down, in the following order, what you would be if you were:

A building

A fabric

A color

A food

A scent

A song

A city

An animal

A period in history

A language

A musical instrument

A form of movement

A chemical

A sound

An element

A work of art

Try to write your answers down instantly, without too much analysis. Go from your gut. Once you have reviewed your answers, take a few moments to write in a journal or talk to someone about the common threads in your choices. Do you see recurring motifs? Or are you diverse and varied? Then you can draw or collage your answers onto a big sheet of drawing paper—your Symbolic Self-Portrait. Or place pictures on a bulletin board, fashion-editor style, if you prefer. If you don't like the way you perceive yourself, realize that your mind is the easiest place to generate transformation, and begin to feed your personal image bank with images that inspire you and represent how you would like to feel about yourself. Maybe you have some fun pictures of yourself as a teenager or young child that you can post to remind yourself of that inner kid who's still inside you, waiting to come out and play. Keep this portrait up where you can see it frequently for a week or two, and notice if it inspires you to make interesting new choices about your appearance— perhaps you'll start to like wearing a fun new color that you wouldn't normally choose.

Appreciation and Gratitude

Appreciation is a great way to experience beauty. Appreciate what you find beautiful in yourself, and encourage that quality to grow. Our minds act like a magnifying glass: whatever we focus on mentally expands. It is a divine law that gratitude for what you have creates the energy to receive more. Try an affirmation when you look in the mirror, such as "I love and approve of myself today." Or be really specific—affirm how you like your smile, or your eyes, and so on. This self-love will help you to focus on the positive, and you will be ready to receive more positive appreciation. By the same token, giving selflessly to others will create more abundant energy in your life. One of the best ways to practice being of service to others is anonymously: try to do one thing for someone else each day without telling anyone about it. This way your actions will be purified by selflessness. It may be tempting to tell others, but this is your ego trying to take credit. Do it for love, not ego.

We can encourage beauty in ourselves by loving others. Volunteer work is a powerful and transformative way to get out of self-consciousness and into helping others. Opportunities for volunteer work abound: check out local senior citizens' centers, animal shelters, Big Brothers and Big Sisters organizations, tutoring or reading to children at the local library, or helping to clean up a beach or a local park. Beautify the world around you and be in touch with the beauty of the divine presence.

Conservation

Maintenance does not seem as dramatic and splashy as creation and death, but it is in fact the bulk of daily existence and life itself. The essence of this book is really about maintenance, and maintenance is the one area where we really can have the most hands-on impact. We can't choose when we're born, and we generally don't choose when we die, but we *can* choose how we live, preserve, and extend or shorten our lives. Maintenance applies not just to our own health and well-being but also to the way we take care of those around us, as well as the planet and its resources. Conserve your energy for what is most important, and watchfully use the resources of the planet.

When we feel our lives are useful and pointed toward a higher purpose, we radiate and embody divine beauty. Being in service is considered to be a high spiritual path in yogic philosophy. No matter who you are or what you do, try to approach your work and life from a place of service. Let this attitude transform your life.

The path of yoga is essentially one of opening the heart. Your changeless and radiant self is always there, waiting to be accessed through many of the practices I have outlined in this book. As we allow our hearts to open, the ability to love is increased. When we love ourselves more deeply, we can also love those around us to a fuller extent. Open the heart to unlock the eternal beauty of the face.

Practicing the Yoga Face techniques of facial relaxation through breath, voice, and yoga, coupled with facial toning through asana and facial exercise, will de-age the face and body, but equally important, these techniques will help uncover the radiant beauty of the spirit, which is a total beauty that is truly ageless.

The beatific, shining face of someone who is happy and in touch with her inner light is truly dazzling. When you smile, it is contagious, and it instantly brightens your features. If you are carrying a mask of worry and fear, becoming more positive will instantly neutralize. A radiant, open heart will give you a clear and sweet face, delighting all who see it.

Be genuinely amiable when you are with others. Never be a "sourpuss." You don't have to laugh boisterously, like a hyena, but don't wear a long face either. Just be smiling, congenial, and kind.

— PARAMAHANSA YOGANANDA*

* From *Inner Reflections*, selections from the writings of Paramahansa Yogananda. Copyright © 2006 Self-Realization Fellowship.

Acknowledgments

I offer gratitude to my teachers: France Nguyen, Peter Rizzo, Alison West, David Life, and Sharon Gannon, all of whom taught me in distinctive ways the true alchemical power of yoga. I extend warm thanks to all my students, whose willingness and enthusiasm helped to birth this book, and who collectively taught me more than I gave.

Thank you to my wonderful husband, Ian Pendleton, who gamely tried the Satchmo as well as the Marilyn . . . with an almost straight face. Thanks to Barbara Ackerman-Kravitz for her nutritional wisdom. I owe much gratitude to Monica Watters for her dermatological, nutritional, and spiritual expertise.

Om shanti to Connie Chan of Levitate Yoga for hosting this workshop in its infancy, and for storing all the mirrors. I owe many thanks to J. Travis and Maryann Donner of the New York Health & Racquet Club for their unflagging faith and excitement. We did it, guys! I owe special gratitude to my literary agent, Margaret Gee. I express my heartfelt appreciation to Michael Ellsberg, for helping this book come to fruition. I am indebted to my editor, Lucia Watson, for her keen insight and enthusiasm. Thanks also to my publisher, Avery.

Thanks to my mother, Karen Gruetter, for modeling ageless beauty, compassion, and joie de vivre. Thanks to Bill Hagen, my father, for exemplifying scholarship and creativity. Thanks to Ursula Heckner-Hagen; her glamour and wit are sources of inspiration.

I am indebted to all the teachers and healers who came before, the ones who offered us this practice; they are the true sources of inspiration and wisdom. I bow to the highest teacher of all:

Om Bolo Sat Guru Bhagavan, Qi Jai
Hari Om Tat Sat

Suggested Reading

Chia, Mantak. *Chi Self-Massage: The Taoist Way of Rejuvenation* (Huntington, New York: Healing Tao Books, 1986).

Chodron, Pema. *Awakening Loving-Kindness* (Boston: Shambhala, 1996).

Coulter, H. David. *Anatomy of Hatha Yoga: A Manual for Students, Teachers, and Practitioners* (Honesdale, Pennsylvania: Body and Breath, 2001).

Danielou, Alain. *Yoga: Mastering the Secrets of Matter and the Universe* (Rochester, New York: Inner Traditions International, 1991).

Iyengar, B. K. S. *Light on Life: The Yoga Journey to Wholeness, Inner Peace, and Ultimate Freedom* (Emmaus, Pennsylvania: Rodale, 2005).

Iyengar, B. K. S. *Light on Yoga* (New York: Schocken, 1976).

Kapit, Wayne, and Lawrence M. Elson. *The Anatomy Coloring Book,* 2nd ed. (Boston: Addison-Wesley, 1993).

Khalsa, Dharma Singh, M.D., and Cameron Sauth. *Meditation as Medicine: Activate the Power of Your Natural Healing Force* (New York: Pocket Books, 2001).

Kushi, Michio. *Your Face Never Lies* (Wayne, New Jersey: Avery, 1983).

Linklater, Kristin. *Freeing Shakespeare's Voice: The Actor's Guide to Talking the Text* (New York: Theater Communications Group, 1992).

Nhat Hanh, Thich. *Being Peace* (Berkeley, California: Parallax, 1987).

Rama, Swami. *Science of Breath: A Practical Guide* (Honesdale, Pennsylvania: Himalayan Institute Press, 1979).

Yogananda, Paramhansa. *Autobiography of a Yogi* (Los Angeles: Self-Realization Fellowship, 1946).

Index

the
yoga
face